Preparing
NURSING
RESEARCH
for the 21st Century

Faye G. Abdellah, R.N., Ed.D., Sc.D., F.A.A.N., Rear Admiral USPHS (Ret) is the former Deputy Surgeon General of the U.S. Public Health Service. She is the recipient of 66 professional and academic honors, including the unique honor of being elected as a Charter Fellow of the American Academy of Nursing. She later served as Vice President and President. Sigma Theta Tau awards include Excellence in Nursing (Kappa, 1983) and the first Presidential Award (1987). The prestigious Allied Signal Award (1989) recognized her pioneering research in aging. In 1992 she received the Institute of Medicine Gustav O. Lienhard Award in recognition of her contributions to the environment and healthier lifestyles.

Dr. Abdellah is the recipient of 10 honorary degrees from universities that have recognized her pioneering work in nursing research and in the development of the nurse scientist; as an international expert on health problems; and for making significant contributions to the health of the nation.

Dr. Abdellah is the author or co-author of more than 150 publications, some translated into six languages.

Recent activities include serving as Sigma Theta Tau's Distinguished Research Fellow (1990–1991); Emily Myrtle Smith Professorship, University of South Carolina, Columbia; and Adjunct Professor of School of Public Health, USC (1990–1991). On March 1, 1993, Dr. Abdellah was appointed Executive Director, (Acting Dean), Graduate School of Nursing, Uniformed Services University of the Health Sciences, Bethesda, Maryland.

Eugene Levine, Ph.D., is currently a consultant on research methodology to a number of organizations, including Georgetown University School of Nursing, the Uniformed Services University of the Health Sciences, and the Indian Health Service of the U.S. Public Health Service (USPHS). Dr. Levine received a B.B.A. from City College of New York, and M.P.A. from New York University, and a Ph.D. in statistics and management from American University. For nearly 30 years he headed the statistical program of the Division of Nursing of the USPHS. In that role he conducted studies on nurse staffing, turnover, productivity, and satisfaction with nursing care. He has authored or co-authored more than 100 journal articles, monographs, and books on his research projects and on research methodology. In 1965 he co-authored with Dr. Abdellah the pioneering textbook *Better Patient Care Through Nursing Research*. He is senior author of a book that presents a comparative analysis of nursing in the United States, Canada, and Great Britain, entitled *Nursing Practice in the UK and North America*.

Preparing
NURSING RESEARCH
for the 21st Century

Evolution, Methodologies, Challenges

Faye G. Abdellah, RN, EdD, ScD, FAAN
Eugene Levine, PhD

with editorial assistance from
Barbara S. Levine, BA

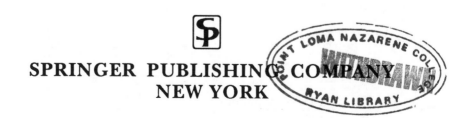

SP

SPRINGER PUBLISHING COMPANY
NEW YORK

Springer Publishing Company, Inc.
536 Broadway
New York, NY 10012-3955

        96 97 98 / 5 4 3 2

Library of Congress Cataloging-in-Publication Data

Abdellah, Faye G.
    Preparing nursing research for the 21st century : evolution,
methodologies, challenges / Faye G. Abdellah, Eugene Levine.
        p.   cm.
    Includes bibliographical references and index.
    ISBN 0-8261-8440-5
    1. Nursing—Research—Methodology.   2. Nursing—Research—United
States.   I. Levine, Eugene.   II. Title.
    [DNLM: 1. Nursing Research—trends—United States.   WY 20.5 A135p
1994]
RT81.5.A26   1994
610.73'072—dc20
DNLM/DLC
for Library of Congress   94–6045
                                                                      CIP

Printed in the United States of America

Contents

Part III   The Impact of Nursing Research on Society

Foreword

As the American health care crisis has loomed larger and larger, I have been steeped in possible solutions, possible reforms to prevent what seemed to be inevitable chaos. It should have come as no surprise how much the contribution of nursing came to my attention in reference to whatever issue I have faced.

Initially, it was obvious that we are a society bent on curative efforts, even when our better judgment should tell us they may be futile. We need to do much more about health problems we can't cure, but for which we can provide care. The contribution of nursing to that issue came frequently to mind.

Long association with some of the underlying dissatisfactions with health care led me to one conclusion: the chief reason other industrialized nations seemed more satisfied with their health care delivery really had less to do with the quality of health care delivered than with the number of primary care providers available to deliver it. We really have a serious shortage—only 29% of our physicians provide primary care, as compared to 54% in Canada, and 70% in the United Kingdom—and the reason we are not closer to chaos is that nurse practitioners, public health nurses, and other health care providers have been doing the job, especially in rural America and inner cities. Humanitarian skills are the hallmarks of the nursing profession, which are supplemented by scientific knowledge and technical skills.

Yet, I had to ask myself how much better this care could have been if more research had been done on the effectiveness of the whole health care system.

Two professions that have served the American people so well in tandem—nursing and medicine—have not really made the best use of available ideas, tools, and philosophies to utilize the contributions of nursing to health care. It is clear that we need better research if health care reform is to be all that it can be.

Health care reform has not always been given high priority by health policy makers. Even if we knew what kind of health care systems were needed, it would take a decade to achieve our goal. Unfortunately, universal and affordable access to health care will not produce a healthy nation by itself. The nursing profession senses this.

Health is not the same as health care. We need a broad enough definition of health to allow us to see how intertwined health is with poverty, greed, and the lack of education—major diseases of our society. Therein lies one of the great contributions that I expect from the profession of nursing. The goals of health care reform are to make health care accessible, of high quality, and of low cost. The material presented by Abdellah and Levine in this book on nursing research for the 21st century will help to achieve these goals.

C. Everett Koop, M.D., Sc.D.
Surgeon General
United States Public Health Service
1981–1989

Preface

The purpose of this book is to share with the readers our assessment of the past and present status of nursing research in order to project its future. We have approached this task from several perspectives. First, each author has been involved in nursing research for over four decades. We have directed a number of large and influential studies in nursing. We wrote the first major textbook in nursing research. Finally, we have held positions in the federal government in which outcomes of nursing studies have been transformed into policy decisions having a major impact on nursing education, practice, and research.

We raise a number of important questions about nursing research in this book and attempt to provide answers based on our best analyses of the direction of the field. What has nursing research achieved in the past 40 years? What have we learned from this research and how will it be applied in the future? Is there an identifiable body of nursing theory? What is the relationship between theory and practice? Are we any closer to developing a nursing science? What methodologies have been used in nursing research and which are the most promising for future studies? Are patients/clients better off because of the results of nursing research? What are areas for future research in nursing?

This book is not a routine textbook on nursing research. Since the appearance of our *Better Patient Care Through Nursing Research* in 1965, the shelves have become filled with an assortment of books on nursing research, including some specializing in one technique or another. The purpose of this book is to present a commentary, in jargon-free and understandable language, on the state of the art of nursing research. It does not contain a detailed explanation of the mechanics of research that so many books have amply provided. Rather than another "how to do it" orientation, we take a more critical and analytical approach, emphasizing "why to do it."

It is our belief that researchers in nursing as well as consumers of nursing research need a sophisticated understanding of how methodology has evolved; why certain methods are used; and what the limitations and strengths of these methodologies are. This increased understanding should provide insights into their structures, purposes, and limitations, affording readers a deeper appreciation of what the methods can and cannot do. This will be useful to consumers of research as well as researchers.

This book brings together in one place discussions that will attempt to answer the following questions:

- What is qualitative research and how can it contribute to nursing research? How does it differ from quantitative research?
- Are randomized clinical trials applicable to nursing? Are there ways of easing the rigid requirements of a controlled study while still obtaining valid results?
- Can meta-analysis be useful in nursing? What are some of the latest approaches to the integration of data in research, such as cross-design synthesis?
- Why are outcome measures important in nursing research? How can measures of health status, functional capability, and quality of life be used in nursing studies?
- What is the state of the art in measurement of the quality of nursing care? How are outcome measures used in evaluation of quality of care? How will the development of clinical practice guidelines help in both the evaluation of quality of care and the design of outcome measures for research? What is the future of quality assurance programs in nursing?
- How can the use of methodologies in nursing research be improved in the future? Is there a trend toward overuse of statistical methodology in nursing studies? What is the real meaning of statistical significance? How does it differ from practical and substantive significance? What are some of the most common mistakes made in using statistical methodology? Is the concept of statistical "power" really important in nursing research? What are the trends in designing cost-effective studies?
- What is the impact of nursing research on health policy formulation? Why is it important to understand this link? What role will nurse researchers play in policy formulation in the future?
- What are the funding strategies for nursing research in the future? What are future priorities? What is the future role of the federal government?

- What have been the major trends in nursing research since its inception? What is nursing research likely to be in the 21st century? What are the trends in educational preparation for nursing research?

The 13 chapters of this book are divided into three sections:

Part I traces the evolution of nursing research from its beginnings as observational studies to the controlled studies of today. The development of quantitative research and the impact of social science research after World War II is described. Major milestones in the growth of nursing research are noted. Professional training issues are discussed.

Part II identifies methodologies that have emerged as the tools of nursing research. Methodologies are critiqued from the point of view of use, overuse, and misuse. The "security bubble" of using methodologies as a cushion is discussed. The distinction between qualitative and quantitative methodology is explained. New approaches with promise for future clinical research in nursing are discussed, including outcomes research, development of clinical practice guidelines, and efficacy and effectiveness research. The extended discussion of the randomized clinical trial assesses its future applicability in clinical nursing research as well as in other types of research in which interventions are evaluated within a research design that attempts to maximize internal and external validity.

Part III discusses the impact of research on health policy formulation and what needs to be done if nursing is to influence the national health agenda. Also discussed are some potential funding strategies for nursing research. Nursing research in the 21st century is examined, including the current gaps and the exciting breakthroughs needed that nurses have to be aware of and become involved in. The career trajectories and educational preparation of nurse researchers and nurse scientists, and the necessary environment that makes for a community of effective nurse scholars, are discussed.

Brief presentations of the historical evolution of nursing research methods are included in each chapter, since we believe that this will promote a better appreciation of the strengths and weaknesses of these methods. The historical perspective will also shed light on current gaps in knowledge that should be addressed by research.

We have attempted to provide clear, concise descriptions and explanations of topics that are often confusing, controversial, or even mysterious. A wide range of topics is covered, some not found in conventional text books on nursing research or only briefly discussed. We believe that our book will fill in some important gaps and will be a very useful source of information and ideas to nurse researchers, and users of research, and all those interested in enhancing their research literacy.

F.G.A.
E.L.

PART I

The Evolution of Nursing Research

Chapter 1

The Early Development of Nursing Research

Nursing research has been influenced by trends in nursing in general. These trends can be categorized into four phases.

The Service Phase

The service phase, influenced by the Nightingale School, began at the turn of the century and lasted from 1900 to 1946. It embodied the belief that nurses should be prepared for a service function.

Nurses were educated predominantly in hospital-based programs in apprentice-type settings during this period. Due to increased demands for nurses and because many nurses during World War II served in the uniformed services (Army, Navy, Air Force, and the U.S. Public Health Service), a large number of practical nurses and nursing aides were trained for employment in hospitals. Thus, nursing became hierarchical, from utilization of nursing aides to baccalaureate-prepared nurses.

In this period registered nurses (RNs) were responsible, without formal preparation, for integrating practical nurses, nursing aides, and orderlies into administration programs. Thus a trend toward improving nursing services through better-prepared managers and administrators began.

During this phase, engineers trained in operations research techniques conducted motion and time studies of nurses in the workplace. Sociologists studied roles and functions of nurses. Nurses frequently helped to collect data, but were not involved in the development or implementation of these studies.

The Academic Phase

In 1948, Esther L. Brown published a strategic blueprint, known as the Brown Report, placing nursing education programs in universities. A national effort was undertaken to implement the recommendations of the Brown Report. Nurses seeking the academic route after 1950 had a choice of graduate majors in administration, supervision, or teaching.

During the academic phase, research focused on curriculum research, teaching methods, and role functions of dean and faculty. One frustration was that, with the exception of psychiatric nursing, there was no support for clinical specialties. The Department of Health, Education and Welfare (now the Department of Health and Human Services) continued this trend in the Nurse Training Act of 1964, which provided support for the preparation of teachers, supervisors, and administrators, but excluded support for advanced preparation in clinical specialties. This gap in support in the face of an obvious need led to the development of the clinical phase.

The Clinical Phase

In the 1960s nurses had to transfer to administrative and academic positions within the profession to achieve recognition and assume a challenging role in nursing. There were many nurses who wanted to advance their careers without abandoning direct patient care, however.

As a result advanced practice nurses began to appear. These nurses are registered nurses who have completed graduate level education (usually at the master's level) and/or are certified in an area of specialization, such as family nurse practitioners who are educated in the provision of integrated primary health care, and available for a wide variety of health care settings. Advanced practice nurses also include certified nurse midwives and nurse anesthetists.

As physician-extender programs developed, the need for clarification of the functions and responsibilities of advanced practice nurses led to the appointment by the Secretary of DHEW of the Committee to Study Extended Roles for Nurses in 1971. The Committee's report included recommendations for acute care and long-term care, thus establishing the parameters of practice for these areas (U.S. Department of Health Education and Welfare, [DHEW] 1971). Critical care nursing and gerontological nursing were next to emerge (Abdellah, 1972).

Nurses during this phase faced two frustrations: 1) a lack of preparation in the basic sciences that could validate nursing practices, and 2) a lack of outcome measures that could be used to document the effects of nursing practices upon patient care. Two decades were to pass before the research on outcome measures and clinical practice guidelines began to emerge in the 1990s.

Impact of Federal Governmental Nurse Leaders

The nursing programs of the U.S. Public Health Service under the leadership of Assistant Surgeon General Lucile Petry Leone, Pearl McIver, and Margaret G. Arnstein stimulated the postwar expansion of nursing services through pilot studies, nursing research, and community health services.

Lucile Petry Leone organized and directed the Cadet Nurse Corps in World War II (1943–45). Pearl McIver guided the development of nursing programs in state and local health departments throughout the United States. Margaret G. Arnstein directed studies of nursing needs and resources that had a major impact on the future supply of nurses. These three leaders were awarded the Mary and Albert Lasker Award in 1955 in recognition of their contributions (American Public Health Association [APHA], 1955).

Surveys and Studies of the Division of Nursing Resources, USPHS

The Division of Nursing Resources, with a modest budget of $95,000 and a small staff, was able to undertake a number of landmark studies to find solutions to postwar nursing problems in hospitals and health agencies. During the years 1949–1955, a number of state surveys of nursing needs and resources were conducted in almost all states. These were short-term projects, funded with small budgets, with the objective of planning practical action programs. They were intended to provide data to assist states in the reorganization and distribution of nursing services as well as in the recruitment and preparation of additional nursing personnel. The surveys were forerunners of action research and laid the ground work for additional intramural studies (Simmons & Henderson, 1964). These surveys, which are still conducted periodically, have become indispensable parts of the effort to maintain a coherent picture and understanding of the dynamics of nursing within the total health system.

In 1954, among the many studies and tools developed by the U.S. Public Health Service's Division of Nursing Resources (now the Division of Nursing) was a cooperative study carried out with the Commission on Nursing of Cleveland to discover the reasons for the understaffing of nursing departments. The study determined the relationship between hours of nursing care and the patient's satisfaction with care (Abdellah & Levine, 1958). Another aspect of the study examined opinions about the care that nurses provided to patients. A byproduct of the study was that it produced an outcome measure— patient satisfaction (Abdellah & Levine, 1957b).

Another important study of this era involved the use of disease classification for nursing planning (Abdellah & Levine, 1954). The basic purpose of this study was to develop a tool for determining the extent to which small hospitals could provide appropriate clinical experiences for students. The methodology consisted of collecting discharge diagnoses of patients in randomly selected hospitals. The diagnoses were then coded and classified into 58 groups representing discrete nursing problems. A similar methodological approach was followed in the development of the problem-oriented medical record more than a decade later. It was also used in the development of diagnosis-related groups (DRGs) (Levine & Abdellah, 1984). These were important steps forward; there was now a standardized and clear reference that could aid the nursing process.

Impact of DRGs: A Watershed Event for Nursing Research

The Tax Equity and Fiscal Responsibility Act of 1982 (Public Law 97–248) and the Social Security Amendments of 1983 (P.L. 98–21) mandated that beginning in October 1983, care for hospitalized Medicare patients would be reimbursed on a flat illness-specific amount established prospectively. The previous system, which reimbursed hospitals after services were rendered, had no incentive for cost containment. The costs incurred included the total expense of each day of care as well as the ancillary services that patients received. Paying hospitals an amount fixed in advance was viewed as a potent mechanism for containing costs of hospital care, which had been escalating since the adoption of the Medicare program in 1965. The prospective payment methodology uses disease classification for the purpose of billing rather than the clinical management of patient care.

The impact of the introduction of DRGs on nursing research was considerable as it brought to light the need for outcome measures specific to nursing research. It stimulated the use of a variety of managed care systems and involved nurses in increased management of patient care. It also stimulated the expansion of the utilization of nurses in noninstitutional care settings, such as home health care. A critical flaw in the DRG method was the omission of a nursing cost component for each of the diagnostic categories. It took almost another decade after the introduction of DRGs for clinical practice guidelines for health care providers that included cost components and outcome measures to become available. The work of Werley, creating a minimum dataset in nursing and defining common terms when applied to DRGs, furthered the identification of a cost component for nursing (Werley & Lang, 1988).

Nursing Research Grants and Fellowships Programs of the Federal Government

In 1955, Congress earmarked $625,000 for nursing research and fellowships that were awarded directly to universities, hospitals, health agencies, or professional associations. These grants and fellowships were directed toward finding ways of improving the quality of nursing care and preparing nurses to undertake research. The research grants program was administered cooperatively by the Division of Nursing Resources (later the Division of Nursing) and the National Institutes of Health (Abdellah, 1970).

The National Center for Nursing Research

In 1986, thirty years after the idea was first proposed by NIH's National Advisory Council, the National Center for Nursing Research (NCNR), was established at the National Institutes of Health. It was authorized by the Health Research Extension Act of 1985 (P.L. 99–158) and established by the Secretary of DHHS in April 1986. Its mandate was "to advance science to strengthen nursing practice and health care that promotes health, prevents disease, and ameliorates the effects of illness and disability."

The placement of NCNR at NIH moved nursing research into a broader based biomedical research environment and facilitated the collaboration between nursing and other research disciplines.

On June 9, 1993, the NCNR was renamed and became the National Institute of Nursing Research, which placed nursing on an equal footing with other NIH Institutes.

Nursing care research is defined as research directed to understanding the nursing care of individuals and groups and the biological, physiological, social, behavioral, and environmental mechanisms influencing health and disease that are relevant to nursing care. Nursing research develops knowledge about health and the promotion of health over the lifespan, care of persons with health problems and disabilities, and nursing actions that enhance the ability of individuals to respond effectively to actual or potential health problems (National Institute of Health, 1989).

The National Institute of Nursing Research is the key organ for funding nursing research grants and contracts. It is now an independent, full fledged institute and partner, as well as a collaborator in biomedical and behavioral research at the National Institutes of Health (NIH).

Recent Milestones in Nursing Research

The establishment of the Agency for Health Care Policy and Research (AHCPR) in December 1988 was another major milestone that has contributed to the development of nursing research. This agency focuses on the development of clinical practice guidelines, outcome measures, and effectiveness research. (AHCPR is discussed in more detail in Chapter 11, pp. 214–216.)

Other Major Milestones

Sigma Theta Tau International

Sigma Theta Tau International was established as an honor society in nursing and for almost six decades has made research grant awards to increase the body of knowledge that is basic to nursing practice. Two examples are the Dissertation Award, initiated in 1989, and the Research Utilization Award Program. The latter is made to an individual or group who has used research as the basis for practice innovation and provided the leadership for utilization of research in clinical practice.

A major accomplishment of Sigma Theta Tau was entering Survey of Nurse Researchers data into a flexible database structure, resulting in the *1990 Directory of Nurse Researchers* (3rd Ed) (Hudgings, 1990).

In 1992, the Virginia Henderson International Nursing Library was established to enhance access to nursing information and knowledge; form electronic communication networks answering nurse researchers; provide a directory of nursing and health care data sources; develop selected nursing databases to facilitate nursing research; provide a structure and classification scheme to organize information about nursing research; and disseminate nursing research funding to the public (Goldstein, 1992).

Sigma Theta Tau's the *Ten Year Plan for Knowledge* focuses on **development, dissemination, and obligation**. Examples of strategies include the communication to lay and professional groups of nursing's significant role in addressing critical issues in health care, and the development of an efficient computerized storage and retrieval system for nursing research and nurse researchers (Sigma Theta Tau International, 1986).

Annual Review of Nursing Research (ARNR)

The publication of the tenth volume of the Annual Review of Nursing Research Series was an important milestone for the scientific nursing community (Fitzpatrick, 1992). The ARNR was the brainchild of Dr. Harriet Werley, who recognized the need to develop an annual integrative critical review of published nursing research. In 1982, Werley's dream came true when she, as first editor, encouraged and supported by the President of the Springer Publishing Company, began to publish the ARNR series. Both editor and publisher believed that the series "could serve as a stimulus for more research."

The purpose of the ARNR is to conduct systematic reviews of research literature; provide guidance to graduate students and faculty in specific nursing fields for research; and to provide critical evaluations for health policy decision makers.

By mandate, the series would be limited to the critical review of *published* research, and only reputable, well-established scholars were invited to contribute. The first volume was published in 1983.

ARNR was the *first* publication to identify "themes" related to nursing practice. Focus was to be on research pertinent to nursing and limited to those studies conducted or co-directed by nurses. Nursing (practice) research was to focus on the individual patient, the family, the environment, and the community as these relate to health. Thus, nurse researchers involved in the development of outcome measures and clinical practice guidelines had a source for publication.

The ARNR series in the 21st century will continue to provide nurse researchers "with an ever-growing role in knowledge development by improving the efficiency with which investigators conduct their literature reviews" and provide scholars with information about promising ideas in nursing research (Stevenson, 1992).

Nursing Research Journals

Because the nursing profession entered the field of research at a relatively late date, the first official nursing research journal appeared only in 1952. Originally sponsored by the National League for Nursing Education and now published by the American Journal of Nursing Company, it was aptly named *Nursing Research,* and was completely devoted to publishing reports of nursing studies and discussions of methodological issues.

It was not until 1966 that another periodical appeared that routinely included reports of nursing studies—the annually published *Nursing Clinics of North America*. The journal, *Image*, sponsored by Sigma Theta Tau, was launched in 1967 to provide a source of scholarly articles on research and other topics. In 1969, the first Canadian research journal began publication, the *Canadian Journal of Nursing Research*.

The decade of the 1970s saw the introduction of several American nursing journals and annuals exclusively devoted to scholarly and research topics: *Research in Nursing and Health* (1978), *Advances in Nursing Science* (1978), the *Western Journal of Nursing Research* (1979), and *Scholarly Inquiry Nursing Practice* (1987). In the United Kingdom, publication of two nursing journals devoted to research and scholarly topics also began during this period: *International Journal of Nursing Studies* (1974) and *Journal of Advanced Nursing* (1976).

The 1980s saw the introduction of several research-oriented publications, including *Applied Nursing Research* (1988), *Nursing Science Quarterly* (1988), *Scholarly Inquiry in Nursing Practice* (1987), and *Journal of Transcultural Nursing* (1989). The 1990s promises to be a prolific decade for nursing research periodicals. So far, two new journals have appeared: *Clinical Nursing Research* (1992) and the interestingly named *Journal of Nursing Measurement* (1993).

Chapter 2

The Growth and Diffusion of Nursing Research through Professional Education

The three phases described in Chapter 1 each identified the need for professional education in the basic sciences, advanced practice (clinical specialties), administration, education research, and historical research. This chapter describes the development of doctoral education—the trajectory leading to careers in nursing research; models and issues in doctoral education; doctoral preparation and research productivity; and the future of doctoral education in research.

Although small-scale research is now widely conducted at the master's level, mainly for training purposes, competence in research in the 21st century will be mandated at the doctoral level for faculty appointments, investigators and for those in leadership and health policy positions. Thus, the emphasis in this chapter is on the doctoral level.

Development of Doctoral Education

Doctoral education for nurses has importance in nursing research and policy decisionmaking. Doctoral education expands and solidifies knowledge in nursing and provides leverage for nurses in securing a policymaking role in the health care system (Grace, 1978).

The initial emphasis of doctoral education in nursing was on preparation of nurse educators (Murphy, 1985). The first doctoral program for nurses was established at Teachers College, Columbia University in 1924 with the Ed. D. degree being awarded to nurses preparing to teach at the college level. Not until the 1950s was the curriculum broadened to include research methodologies for those wishing to pursue a career in research. The first Ph.D. program in nursing was established in 1934 at the School of Education at New York University (Werley & Lang, 1988).

Grace (1978) described three evolutionary stages of the development of doctoral preparation for nurses. The first stage (1926–1959) focused on functional specialists to prepare nurses to teach at college levels. The second stage (1960–1969) was the nurse scientist era in which nurses obtained doctoral preparation in disciplines related to nursing. This effort was spearheaded by the establishment of Nurse Scientist Training Programs funded by the Division of Nursing and the National Center for Health Services Research, USPHS. The Division also funded predoctoral and postdoctoral research fellowships. The third stage emerged in the 1970s with the awarding of doctorates in nursing, namely the DNS, DNSc, and the ND.

In 1971, Matarazzo and Abdellah sought to identify the directions of doctoral education in nursing. The first American study program awarding the Doctor of Philosophy degree was established at Yale University in 1861. It took almost 100 years for a sufficient knowledge base to be developed so that a substantive Ph.D. in nursing could be offered. The availability of federal funds for doctoral preparation in recent years has had a major impact in increasing the number of nurses obtaining doctoral preparation (Marriner-Tomey, 1990).

Paradoxically, despite the large body of scientific knowledge that exists today, there are severe inadequacies in the quality and availability of health care for Americans. Much needed is the development of doctoral programs for nurses and in nursing directed toward building and applying the scientific knowledge base from which high-quality nursing practice results. The challenge for doctoral education in nursing is to move nursing theories and knowledge from a descriptive level to a practical level (Grace, 1989).

Grace (1978) and others have expressed the view of many nurse leaders that nursing needs nurses with doctorates in nursing, education, and related disciplines. There has been much discussion about the doctoral degree itself, and whether a Ph.D., DNS, or ND should be in nursing only. The Ph.D. program was thought appropriate for the nurse researcher who wishes to develop nursing theories, and the DNS and ND programs designed for clinicians who test nursing theories in a broader clinical context (Fields, 1988).

Models and Issues in Doctoral Education

The evolvement of doctoral programs has brought to the surface a number of problems and issues (Grace, 1989):

- There has been a lack of agreement on the substantive content of doctoral programs.
- Newly graduated nurse scientists brought to their work traditions and biases learned as doctoral students in related fields. Those from the natural sciences brought the research mentorship process. Those from the behavioral sciences mastered a body of theoretical knowledge and worked under the mentorship of faculty to do independent research.
- The newly emerging clinical specialty professional doctorate was controversial.
- Doctoral programs became "loaded" with course requirements in an attempt to integrate the sciences into nursing.
- Almost all nursing doctorates were molded into a research doctorate.
- The overload of courses and advising students on their research left faculty little time to do their own research.
- Conversely, the time faculty had to spend on research reduced the time available to spend on teaching, practice, and service.
- Leadership, both in practice and education, became threatened.
- Focus of inquiry at the doctoral level had no resemblance to future employment situations (Williams, 1989).

The central question is how to design a doctoral program that meets the needs and expectations of researchers, expert clinicians, health policy experts, administrators, teachers, ethicists, and historians. Grace (1989) proposes three models to meet these diverse needs:

The Research Doctorate
(Ph.D. or Ed.D., With a Research Focus)

The goal is to prepare competent researchers with a foundation built on the generalist base of basic nursing education. Emphasis of the research doctorate is on research. Key to the success of this model is to have faculty oriented to research who can serve as mentors.

The Clinical/Applied Doctorate (DNS)

This model builds on a clinical specialization base with the primary goal of preparing advanced practitioners/applied researchers.

The Professional Doctorate (ND)

This model is usually a postbaccalaureate first professional degree in nursing. After completing the professional doctorate, those wishing to pursue a career in research or advanced applied research would enter a postbasic program such as a DPH program (Fitzpatrick, 1987).

Doctoral Preparation and Research Productivity

Do nurses with doctorates go on to conduct research? A study conducted by Farren (1991) found that research productivity is influenced by the following factors:

- *Participation in faculty research.* This factor was found to be most significant, as it reinforces the importance of academic mentoring in developing research skills (Anema & Byrd, 1991). The mentoring relationship enables the doctoral student to benefit from serving as an assistant to a faculty member actively engaged in research (Davidhizar, 1988).
- *Importance to nursing.* Regardless of dissertation topic, doctoral graduates do pursue research interests important to nursing.
- *Achievement.* The holders of doctoral degrees such as the Ph.D. or DNS were found to be research achievers (Farren, 1991).

- *Support*. Employer support for research, including released time, was very beneficial.
- *Collaboration* with peers.
- *Availability* of *library resources*.
- Availability of *computer services*.
- *Access* to research populations.

Do doctoral graduates meet job expectations of employers? According to Fitzpatrick (1991), the doctoral graduate who is well prepared in research methodology and capable of independent research has an increased chance of succeeding in the workplace by meeting the demands of the employer. Moreover, the dissertation can be helpful in preparing the graduate for the working world if it addresses a substantive area in nursing, particularly if it results in a publication (Baun, 1987), thereby bringing the author's name to the attention of the reader and potential employers.

Those guiding the careers of nurse scientists should encourage them to consider a postdoctoral program before accepting an academic position. Interactions with other nurses pursuing postdoctorates can help prepare the nurse scientist for the real world (Williams, 1986). By assisting and interacting with a group of researchers with similar research goals, the prospective researcher is helped to acquire an ever-broadening content of scientific and research knowledge.

Because of demands in the clinical situation, employers seek to fill the position of clinical nurse researcher in hospitals and universities. The clinical nurse researcher needs an opportunity to test nursing theory and conduct and apply nursing research (Dennis, 1991). Doctoral students and graduates must have experience in implementing a research role within a variety of settings, including hospital organizations, nursing homes, ambulatory care settings, and home health agencies, in order to understand more completely the research process.

Doctoral graduates wishing to enter the political arena can find no better experience than working as a staff intern at state, regional, and federal governmental agencies. The experience of researching, interviewing consumers, and drafting proposed legislation can involve the doctoral graduate in the process of health policy formulation, thus providing not only an inside view, but insight into the political process as it affects health care.

Environment—A Critical Factor in Research Productivity

The structural elements in a positive nursing research environment are (Pranulis, 1985):

- Competency in research skills;
- Research valued as a desirable outcome;
- Time for faculty to engage in research;
- Faculty research activities compatible with organizational mission;
- Support to seek extramural funding; and
- A psychosocial climate supportive to research.

Holzemer and Chambers (1988) examined the contextual effects of the educational environment on faculty research productivity and found that faculty who spent more time on research were more productive in research. Doctoral programs with highly productive faculty had more such faculty who served as role models, i.e., doing research that could be attributed to an individual. Also, individuals who perceived their environment positively were more productive.

A critical factor was the existence of a collaborative model of mentorship. The model is described as role-specific modeling/teaching and as professionally stimulating. The productive environment provided multiple research activities (Williams & Blackburn, 1988).

The collaborative research model is a cooperative effort among peers, with multiple researchers focusing on a project. Collaborative research is characterized as interagency (members employed at different institutions) or intra-agency (collaboration among members of the same institution) (Cole & Slocumb, 1990).

Another positive influence is a research environment in which doctoral faculty make up a community of scholars. Such a community assures that there exists a "critical mass" of individuals who meet the criteria of scholarship. There also exists a sociological conceptualization of community. Thus, faculty share common traditions and research interests, and a system of informal interdependent relationships exists (Lenz, 1989). Faculty should be encouraged to establish research networks and supportive research teams, encouraging the initiation of research projects as well as publishing the results.

A positive research environment was found to be one in which productivity of research was high; there were authored or co-authored papers with mentors; and less time was spent in teaching and more in administration (Megel, Langston, & Creswell, 1988).

An innovative approach being used by the Department of Veterans Affairs is the establishment of a postdoctoral research fellowship for preparation of clinical researchers to develop research skills and conduct studies under the mentorship of clinical investigators. The goal is to prepare independent clinical investigators (Lawson, 1989).

Strategies to Prepare Doctoral Graduates for Job Expectations

- Provision of research experiences, faculty mentorships in research, and socialization for scholarship;
- Integration of the teaching and research roles of the faculty;
- Faculty serving as referees to provide opportunities for dialogue;
- Encouragement of postdoctoral study under the mentorship of established scientists; and
- Helping doctoral students to set realistic long-term career goals (Ketefian, 1991).

Research scholarship is lifelong learning, sharing, communicating, building on a sound foundation, and linking the research experience to realistic job expectations and health care policy decisionmaking.

Doctoral Education—Preparing for the 21st Century

It is to doctoral graduates that nursing will look for the creative study and testing of the theories of the science of nursing (Downs, 1988). The future of doctoral education in nursing will be shaped by the needs of society, trends in health care systems, and the needs of the profession. One has only to review the report of the U.S. Department of Health and Human Services, (1990), *Promoting Health, Preventing Disease: Year 2000 Objectives for the Nation*, to realize how much doctoral education will be influenced by the priorities specified in the national health agenda. These priorities also will influence the future research agenda, and the two are closely related.

There is little to document actual differences between research and professional doctorates. Meleis (1988) suggests specifying indicators and criteria to differentiate between professional and research doctorates. The content for research doctorates could be organized around conceptual areas such as environment and health, self-care and recovery, and health promotion. The content for professional doctorates could be structured around clinical practice divisions. Successful doctoral programs in the 21st century will be those that focus on substantive issues that are significant for society and the profession.

The challenge of the future for doctoral education is to bring the resources of nursing scholars and the university into a mutually beneficial relationship (Downs, 1978, 1988). The focus of nursing research must be to provide information to guide and improve nursing practice. Nursing research findings can be used to affect health policy at state, regional, and national levels if guided effectively and presented successfully. An objective of doctoral programs should be to promote the commitment of students to use nursing science to affect health care policy (Hinshaw, 1988a). It is an absolute necessity that nursing research findings be communicated beyond the nursing research community in order to reach the attention of health policy makers, otherwise not much will come of it beyond its immediate use in nursing practice.

Hinshaw suggests a collaborative model of research that links nurse scientists with clinicians, health policy makers, and administrators. Presentation of research findings in understandable language can help this linkage.

The 21st century will see much more emphasis on postdoctoral education as a requirement for academic and research positions. Collaborative research will prove to be an effective model for influencing professional colleagues and health policy makers.

A national survey of 439 deans and directors of baccalaureate and higher degree programs were queried about current need and funding capability of researchers prepared with five different foci: psychosocial processes, biophysical processes, health care delivery systems and administration, education, and methodology and instrumentation. They concluded that diverse foci for both current and future researchers was indicated (Sherwen, Bevil, Adler, & Watson, 1993).

PART II

Nursing Research Methodologies and How They are Used

Chapter 3
Trends in Methodologies

Evolution of Research Methodologies

As a field of research, nursing has engaged in a wide variety of methodological applications; few fields offer as much methodological diversity. Applications range from qualitative methods such as ethnography and phenomenology to the highly quantitative techniques of multivariable analysis.

The methodologies of early nursing studies were comparatively simple. Data were mostly collected through field surveys, and the analyses were uncomplicated. Such modest beginnings are true of all research.

Advances in research methodology were greatly assisted by the development of statistics as an analytical methodology. Early uses included analysis of vital events such as births, deaths, and the resultant population changes. But it was not until the publication of R.A. Fisher's classic book, *The Design of Experiments*, in 1935 that the application of statistical techniques to quantitative research really moved forward. Techniques for evaluating causal relationships such as the analysis of variance were greatly advanced by Fisher and other statisticians. In the field of psychological testing, the various techniques of multivariable analysis such as factor analysis were refined and expanded in response to the need for tools to measure aptitudes and abilities of World War II soldiers and veterans by the Department of War. The war was indeed a major stimulant to research methodology development (Cronbach, 1970; Stouffer, Suchman, DeVinney, Star, & Williams, 1949,1950).

Additionally, sampling methodology, an important tool for scientifically selecting research subjects in quantitative research, became increasingly sophisticated after World War II. Today, studies are conducted with small numbers of subjects with assurance that the sample will yield good data economically. Even the decennial United States Census of Population and Housing uses a sample to obtain data on detailed socioeconomic characteristics.

The computer has had a profound effect on the use of statistical methodology in quantitative research. Not only can data be processed more quickly and more cost-effectively, but the analytical power of the methodology has increased to a degree undreamt of when nursing research was in its infancy. Advances are especially marked in multivariable analysis, where powerful modern computers make it possible to examine hundreds of variables simultaneously.

What are Research Methodologies?

The term "methodology" is widely used in research. In its broadest sense it includes the various processes and procedures used to carry out a research project. To be considered scientific, methodology must be orderly, structured, and produce accurate and consistent data. In essence, it should facilitate the search for valid knowledge, the essential purpose of scientific research (Kaplan, 1964).

There are three main areas of methodology in research:

- Research design;
- Data collection; and
- Data analysis

Research design is the overall plan for conducting a research project. Prepared prior to the study, it addresses the aims and purposes of the research, hypotheses or research questions, organization and structure of data collection including introduction of study subjects into the research and safeguarding their rights, and the degree of control by the researcher over all aspects of the research, particularly data collection. The many types of research design extend from highly controlled laboratory experiments to uncontrolled surveys in natural-setting field studies. The researcher chooses the design best suited to the purposes of the study and the research questions to be answered. Resources available for the research also influence the design, especially the amount of time and money available.

Data collection refers to the methods for gathering research data. This includes data-collection instruments to be used—questionnaires and other types of "pencil and paper" tools and mechanical instruments for making measurements, as well as the unstructured tools used in qualitative research. Data collection methodology also includes selection of study subjects, sampling techniques, if any, and the ways of processing data for analysis.

Data analysis includes the many techniques for summarizing and testing data in order to answer the research questions. Since the advent of the computer, an extensive array of analytical tools have become available to examine quantitative data in great detail. The speed, accuracy, and relatively low cost of computer manipulations of data have resulted in the problem of "over-kill" in data analysis, to be addressed later.

Research Approaches

Until recently, research was mostly conducted with quantitative methods. In the past twenty years, however, qualitative methods have been increasingly employed in nursing research. Discussions of methodology use the terms "quantitative" and "qualitative" to distinguish different approaches to research; a trend, incidentally, that has not taken place in related fields, such as medical and health services research, which remain almost completely quantitative. It appears that the subject matter of nursing is congenial to the qualitative approach.

Thus, the term "research approach" can be used to describe a *set* of methods and techniques for designing a study and collecting and analyzing data: quantitative data in quantitative research, and qualitative data in qualitative research. Moreover, the quantitative/qualitative dichotomy implies more than different methods and techniques for conducting research. There are significant conceptual and contextual as well as philosophical differences in the two approaches that will be discussed. In other words, while some of the same research techniques such as content analysis may, be used by these different approaches, the purpose and content as well as the total epistemological foundations of the two are different.

Impact of Methodological Advances on Nursing Research

Advances in methodology have been beneficial to nursing research. Studies reported in the literature of nursing research cover the entire gamut of research methodology. This diversity reflects the wide-ranging subject matter of nursing studies which have embraced the academic disciplines of sociology, psychology, anthropology, physiology, public administration, economics, and engineering.

It is instructive to compare articles in the first issues of *Nursing Research* (launched in 1952) to those published currently. The early issues were replete with descriptive studies of nurses based on simple questionnaires and containing minimal analysis. The content of current issues seems light-years away from the early ones in terms of methodological and analytical variety and sophistication.

Moreover, unlike the early efforts, researchers now attempt to apply research findings to advance the scientific basis of nursing through model and theory development. In addition, there are today about a dozen journals and monographs devoted to reporting nursing research and to discussion of nursing models and theories. That the technique of meta-analysis is being increasingly applied to the critical review and integration of multiple studies in nursing shows not only that nursing research has flourished as to number of completed studies, but has made notable improvements in the quality of research methodologies employed (Brown, 1991).

But progress has not taken place without some undesirable aspects. Sometimes so much effort is placed on the analytical side of the research process that insufficient attention is given to the quality of data. Data quality—reliability, validity, and relevance—is of primary importance to the whole research effort. Some researchers apply highly complex techniques to poor data in the belief that such techniques will compensate for its deficiencies. Unfortunately, it usually does not work. As the venerable adage says, "garbage in, garbage out" (GIGO).

Then, too, computers with their wonderful capability to analyze huge masses of data in an instant, play a role in and indeed may be the prime cause of GIGO. It may seem impressive for a research report to show page after page of multiple regression coefficients or F-ratio values, but the question "What is their *substantive* significance above and beyond their *statistical* significance?" is of paramount importance. If, for example, a 2% difference between two summary measures is found to be statistically significant, the important question is, "What meaningful impact on the real world does this small difference have?"

Because the computer makes it quick and easy to run the statistical tests so commonly used in quantitative research, some test results will turn out to be statistically significant by chance alone. The laws of probability state that there is always a small chance of falsely obtaining a significant result in repeated tests; this is known as the Type I error.

Although some early nursing studies now seem simplistic and superficial, the absence of computers and other tools, as well as scarcity of money to conduct research, did force these researchers to spend considerable time on planning how their data should be collected, analyzed, and interpreted. This put a more individualistic and, perhaps, a more creative stamp on research than is often found today when the computer is expected to do some of the "thinking." This need to conserve resources also motivated researchers to avoid trivial topics. Today, the availability of greater methodological and financial resources has resulted in a bewildering array of research content in nursing. Consequently, a fairly large number of studies have contributed little of significance to the advancement of knowledge.

Summary of Trends In Nursing Research Methodologies

Although nursing research has become more varied and sophisticated since the early studies, there have been no fundamental changes in the way research has been conducted with the exception of more emphasis on qualitative research. A summary of the major trends in nursing research methodology reveals the following. *First*, the six major components of the research process have remained essentially unchanged. They are:

- Statement of the research problem, questions, objectives and purposes;
- Determination of the overall research design or plan: the structure and process for conduct of the study;
- Delineation of the study population and a method for selecting subjects for participation in the research;
- Method for collecting, processing, and analyzing research data; and
- Method for interpreting, disseminating, and utilizing research results.

Second, although research designs have become more elaborate and more efficient in controlling extraneous variables, the basic characteristics of the major designs—experimental, quasi-experimental, non-experimental—have remained essentially unchanged. The use of control groups and placebos to protect against extraneous variables is not new, even though some current writings in the research literature would make it seem so. The impact of uncontrolled variables on research data was identified long ago when, for example, results of industrial engineering studies conducted in the Hawthorne plant of the Western Electric Company were analyzed (Landsberger, 1958; Roethlisberger & Dickson, 1939).

Third, although data collection methodology has become considerably modernized through use of electronic technology, data collection techniques—questionnaires, interviews, participant observation—have not changed significantly. Tools of measurement have improved as more precise instruments have become available, but the fundamental principles of measurement, including concepts of validity and reliability, have remained constant.

Fourth, statistical methods for analyzing quantitative research data, although more versatile and informative today, due largely to the availability of powerful computers, still rest on the same theoretical underpinnings developed by Pearson, Neyman, Yule, Fisher, and others.

Fifth, in the broadest sense, the purposes for undertaking research are varied. The major ones are to:

- Add to fundamental knowledge about a subject;
- Test a theory;
- Solve a problem;
- Develop a new product, procedure, or program; and
- Evaluate a product, procedure, or program.

Because research methodologies are chosen in accordance with the research purpose, studies with similar purposes often use similar methodologies. If, for example, fundamental knowledge about a subject is being sought, an unstructured, nonquantitative approach in a natural setting may well be a useful methodological approach. In such a study data will be collected through observation or open-ended interviews. If the objective is to evaluate whether one way of carrying out a nursing procedure is more effective than another, a more tightly controlled research design is needed. Data for this study might be obtained from use of a measuring instrument that provides a valid and reliable quantitative measure of what constitutes a "better" way of carrying out the procedure.

The Role of Small Studies

Although the trend in nursing research has been toward greater elaboration and complexity, there is much need for studies conducted at all levels, including small, simple studies that can be conducted by a single researcher with modest resources. There are many research topics that could be addressed without recourse to "heavy-duty" methodology and the involvement of large samples. The infatuation with the concept of statistical "power" has led to an increase in sample size, considerably adding to the cost of studies. As some qualitative researchers have demonstrated, many valuable findings have been produced from small samples using simple techniques. Bigger is not necessarily better. Esoteric and overly complicated methodology cannot substitute for well-designed, creatively conducted research on meaningful topics.

In the chapters that follow, the major nursing research methodologies and approaches will be discussed in detail. The emphasis will be on methodologies that have the greatest relevance for future nursing research. One objective of the discussion will be to clarify the purposes and uses of the methodologies and critique the tendencies to misuse or overuse them. The final chapter will offer advice on how the use of these methodologies can be improved in future nursing research.

Chapter 4

Quantitative Research

Introduction

Labeling research as "quantitative" or "qualitative" is a recent development. In the past practically all research in nursing was quantitative, so there was no need for any qualifying terminology; research and quantitative research were interchangeable terms. Even today most nursing studies use quantitative methodology, an emphasis likely to continue. Perhaps the most appropriate terminology should be *research* and *qualitative research*, the latter designating studies in which the methodology is entirely qualitative.

In any case, this chapter proposes to discuss *quantitative* research: what it is, how it is used in nursing research, and how it can be more productively used in the future. The next chapter will discuss qualitative research. Subsequent chapters will address some specific areas of what is largely quantitative research including clinical trials, outcome measures, and meta-analysis.

This chapter will not present an exhaustive discussion of quantitative research, as many journal articles and books in nursing and in other fields offer comprehensive presentations of this subject. The purpose here is to offer some observations that might provide fresh insights on this well-traversed topic.

What is Quantitative Research?

A simple definition of quantitative research is research in which *quantitative* data on *variables* are collected and analyzed. Variables denote specific characteristics, traits, or properties of humans, animals, or things. Variables can be classified as *qualitative* if they describe properties with different levels, types, or kinds that are differentiated qualitatively, in words, as, for example, eye color. By contrast, the variation in *quantitative* variables is described quantitatively, in numbers. In quantitative research, both qualitative and quantitative variables yield numerical data through the use of measurement scales. Qualitative variables are measured by two types of qualitative scales: *nominal* scales of ungraded categories such as political affiliation (Democrat, Republican, other), and *ordinal* scales of graded categories (small, medium, large). Quantities are generated for qualitative scales by *counting* the number of study subjects in each category. Thus, qualitative scales are also called *enumeration* scales. They yield *frequency data* analyzed by *nonparametric* statistical techniques, a somewhat misleading term, because some of these techniques are applied to "parameters" (summary measures) such as relative frequencies and medians.

Quantitative variables are measured by numerical scales called *interval* and *ratio* scales. The difference between these two scales is that an interval scale does not have a true zero point, while a ratio scale does, so that differences in points on the ratio scale are proportional to each other. The scale to measure body temperature is an example of an interval scale, whereas the variable weight is a ratio scale. Quantitative variables are frequently measured by mechanical instruments. These are generally more reliable than the "pencil and paper" instruments used to measure qualitative variables. Moreover, the parametric techniques for analyzing quantitative variables are more versatile and sensitive than nonparametric techniques.

Thus, quantitative research deals with both qualitative and quantitative variables and treats them both numerically. Qualitative research, for the most part, deals only with qualitative variables in a non-numeric way. A major distinction between the two types of research is the role of *statistical methodology*: all-important for quantitative research, negligible or nonexistent for qualitative research. Statistical methodology pervades each step of the research process in quantitative research.

Evolution of Quantitative Nursing Research

The history of quantitative nursing research is essentially the history of nursing research. Early research in nursing and hospitals was mostly quantitative, which set the pattern for the future. Among her many achievements Florence Nightingale was a quite competent statistician. Her studies of hospital performance were filled with quantitative data (Nightingale, 1858, 1861). One of the earliest nursing studies conducted in the United States was contained in the report of the Committee for the Study of Nursing Education (1923). This was largely a quantitative survey of schools of nursing and the various fields in which nurses worked.

Until the first qualitative studies appeared in the early 1960s, all of nursing research was quantitative research. Even today at least 90% of nursing studies are quantitative. This emphasis is not surprising. Quantitative methods dominate most fields of research, anthropological research and areas related to anthropology being the most notable exceptions. Why is this so? Because research and quantification have a symbiotic relationship. Quantification does facilitate research in a number of ways: it promotes objectivity, enhances the efficiency of data aggregation, permits a variety of analytical techniques to be applied to the data, and facilitates dissemination of study findings. Some believe that without quantification there can be no research. Others say, less sweepingly, that without quantification there can be no *explanatory* research, only descriptive research.

In nursing, research progressed from quantitative descriptive studies of individual variables to quantitative explanatory studies of relationships among variables. Abdellah and Levine (1957a) introduced multivariable analysis into nursing research by applying the technique of multiple regression to analyzing the relationship of nursing time to patient satisfaction.

Today, entire books are devoted to the statistical analysis of multiple variables in nursing research (Volicer, 1984). Moreover, nursing research has shifted away from studies of nurses to studies of nursing, namely clinical nursing, as titles of studies supported (1992) by the federal government's National Center for Nursing Research (now National Institute of Nursing Research) revealed. A few recently funded studies, selected at random, suggest a focus on the quantitative relationship among variables as well as a clinical orientation (National Center for Nursing Research, 1992c):

- Chronic memory loss: Home vs. community interventions;
- Accuracy of substituted judgements in terminal illness;
- Nursing's impact on quality-of-life outcomes in elders;
- Coping with head and neck surgery and hospital stay;
- Falls: A predictive model of risk;
- Patient's knowledge and use of legal advance directives; and
- Mother-child interactions and adaptation of toddlers.

As nursing research has progressed from the descriptive to the explanatory, the complexity of quantitative analytical techniques has increased. A recent review of a book on quantitative techniques took the authors to task for spending only a few pages on a discussion of multivariate analysis of variance, a somewhat arcane technique that has found its way into nursing research (Lenz & Soeken, 1992). As studies of relationships among variables have increased, techniques of multivariable analysis are now routinely employed. A study of the impact of AIDS education used such techniques as analysis of variance, analysis of covariance, log linear analysis, and logistic regression analysis (Nyamathi, Leake, Flaskerud, Lewis, & Bennett, 1993). The ordinary summary measures, such as means and standard deviations, that often composed the entire repertoire of analytical tools in earlier studies have been buried under an avalanche of chic methodology.

In addition, more highly quantitative research designs are being used today; for example, in clinical trials. The evolution of nursing research can thus be characterized as a trend toward an intensification of quantification and greater use of more high-powered statistical techniques. To offset this trend there has been growing interest in the nonquantitative approaches of qualitative research.

Statistical Methodology Defined

What is Statistics?

The discipline of statistics has been defined in a number of ways. In one definition statistics are simply numerical facts. In the methodological sense statistics is a body of methods and techniques for obtaining, organizing, analyzing, and interpreting numerical facts. In another definition statistics is a "body of methods for making decisions when there is uncertainty arising from the incompleteness or the instability of the information available" (Wallis & Roberts, 1965, p. 26).

It should be well understood that in research, statistics is not an end in itself, but a means to an end. It is *not a body of substantive knowledge*, but a research methodology linked to a specific content area. Statistics is an end unto itself only to theorists and methodologists who design statistical techniques. In some projects the statistical methodology seems to dominate the study as an end in itself rather than, as Wallis and Roberts have said, to help make good decisions from the assembled data. Many studies are so full of complicated statistical formulas and obstruse data that the *substantive* meaning of the findings is lost. The fascination with esoteric techniques such as *multivariate analysis of variance and discriminant analysis*, to name just a few, has resulted in studies in which the techniques drive the research, rather than being subsidiary and supportive.

Statistics as the Study of Variation

R. A. Fisher, whom many consider the leading figure in the development of statistical methodology, defined statistics in his classic textbook, *Statistical Methods for Research Workers*, (1925) as the study of variation. This is a deceptively simple, but very wise definition. Basically, without variation there would be no data for quantitative research because there would be no variables. Without quantitative data there is no need for statistical methodology. For example, if all diseases were eliminated and there was only one cause of death—old age—there would be no need for the *International Classification of Diseases* and no variables called disease or cause of death. If people's temperatures remained constant at 98.6 degrees regardless of their state of health, there would be no temperature statistics, and one of the most frequently used variables in clinical research would be eliminated. If all people weighed the same, not only would another important clinical research variable be lost, but the impact on society would be enormous: food, clothing, and diet fads, to name just a few areas.

In the real world everything varies; and some things more than others. What may seem invarying on close examination may exhibit much variability. To the naked eye different tissue samples may look identical, but under a microscope may show great dissimilarity. The sole purpose of measuring instruments is to detect variability. The more refined the instrument the greater is its ability to detect fine differences. How much refinement is needed in order to detect small differences depends on how clinically significant the small differences are. It is hard to conceive of a research problem in which a difference in a patient's temperature smaller than one-tenth of a degree—98.60 compared to 98.61, for example—would be important.

Not only does everything vary in terms of a single characteristic, but most objects possess a multiplicity of variables. The number of variables in humans may be almost infinite, limited only by the availability of instruments to measure them. A voluminous set of physiological, biological, sociological, psychological, and anthropological variables are available for use in addressing a huge number of hypotheses and questions of interest. To illustrate, suppose we were interested in measuring the response of elderly persons to the interventions of home health nurses. Response could be measured in many ways, either by a single variable, such as whether the person is taking medications correctly, or by a set of variables in a unified dimension, such as activity status measured by functional capabilities in walking, eating, communicating, personal hygiene, etc., or by a multidimensional index that combines measures of self-care capability, functional capabilities, mental status, and nursing and medical evaluation.

Measurement of variability underlies much of statistical methodology. In descriptive statistics, the usual procedure is to compute a summary measure by combining individual measures. A common summary measure is an average, such as a mean or a median, that represents the central value among the individual measures. An average is not completely informative without an accompanying measure of variation of the values of individual measures such as the range or standard deviation. It is more informative to state that the mean age of employed registered nurses in the United States is 37 years of age and ranges from 18 to 80 years than to report only the mean, and thus convey an impression that all RNs have yet to reach middle age.

Variation is important in the methodological procedure known as *statistical inference* in which a statistical measure is generalized beyond the boundaries of the study: from a sample (the study subjects) to a larger group (the population). For each summary measure obtained from a sample, a *standard error* can be computed by dividing the measure of variation of the individual sample values by the square root of the number of sample measures. The value of the sample summary measure, plus and minus the standard error (usually 2 standard errors), is called the *confidence interval*, the range of values around the sample summary measure within which the population value lies.

Thus, the standard error is a measure of the variation attributable to sampling—the sampling error.

Standard errors can be calculated for *differences* in the values of summary measures for different samples as in the difference in values of outcome measures between control and treatment groups in an experiment. Analysis of the extent to which this difference exceeds the standard error of the difference is called a *test of statistical significance*. When a statistically significant difference is found, the inference is that the sample summary measures came from different populations.

The measurement of variability is important in the statistical analysis of the relationship among variables in using techniques such as correlation and regression analysis. *Multiple regression* analysis measures the dependence of one variable, the *dependent* variable, on a set of variables, the *independent* or "causal" variables. Calculation of the variances of the measurements of the variables is important to *regression* analysis as it is of *analysis of variance* (ANOVA), perhaps the most widely used technique of statistical analysis, and in its multivariable version, *multivariate analysis of variance* (MANOVA). The whole idea of ANOVA is to measure variability and allocate it to different sources.

A quantitative researcher must be aware of variability in data from two standpoints: measuring it and controlling it. Measurement of variability is important *descriptively*, in revealing the spread of the measures, and *evaluatively*, in determining the significance of differences among measures. Controlling variability is important in explanatory studies in minimizing the impact of extraneous variables on the variables of interest. The identification and control of variability is accomplished through study design and statistical procedures.

Evolution of Statistical Methodology

Numbers and measurement and tabulation of statistical data go back in history to Biblical times and the early Egyptians and Greeks. But statistics as a comprehensive and systematic analytical methodology, and particularly as a methodology for conducting controlled studies such as experiments, originated in this century. Credit is usually given to John Graunt for taking an important step in establishing statistics as a methodology for explaining as well as describing phenomena. In 1662 Graunt published a book entitled *Natural and Political Observations made upon the Bills of Mortality*, in which he presented an interpretation of biological and social phenomena based on numbers of births and deaths in London during the years 1604 to 1661 (Newman, 1956). His report was a first attempt at the analytical use of statistics, and helped launch the field of vital statistics.

Thirty years after Graunt's report the astronomer Edmund Halley, among his many other notable achievements, described a methodology to predict life expectancy from statistics on deaths. Halley's approach is still used for determining life insurance rates and projecting future population.

Until the 20th century the major use of statistics was in the field of vital statistics and demography, and not as a comprehensive research tool. It may be surprising to note that statistical methodology was *not* used by such eminent scientists as Galileo, Faraday, Boyle, Galton, and Pasteur in conducting their experiments. Considering their achievements, it must be assumed that they possessed an intuitive sense of how to avoid the pitfalls in research that statistical methodology was later developed to address.

A further contribution to the development of statistics as a tool for conducting research was made by the mathematicians who provided the probability models upon which important areas of statistical analysis depend. One of the earliest contributors was Bernoulli, a contemporary of Graunt and Halley, whose theorem, known as the Law of Large Numbers and published posthumously in 1713, is still of great importance to probability theory. Later mathematicians, such as Poisson, Markoff, Tchebycheff, and De Moivre also advanced the mathematical foundations of statistical methodology.

Perhaps the three key figures in the development of statistical theory and methodology for use in quantitative research in the social sciences were the British scholars Frances Edgeworth, Karl Pearson, and Ronald A. Fisher. Edgeworth (1881) wrote extensively on the application of mathematics to social problems. Pearson, whose writings began at the end of the 19th century, made major contributions to the analysis of correlated variables, a technique that plays such an important role in explanatory research (Pearson, 1896, 1904). Contemporaries of Pearson, including Yule and Student (Pseudonym of W.S. Gosset), also contributed to the advancement of statistical theory.

Fisher's contributions were very broad. As a member of the famous Rothamsted Experimental Station in England after World War I, he pioneered in the application of statistical methodology to the design of experiments in agriculture, genetics and other fields. Fisher showed how statistical theory and methodology can be used in experimental research. In his classic book, *The Design of Experiments* (1935), he explained how statistical techniques can be applied to all research in which variables are measured quantitatively to enhance the internal and external validity of the findings.

Following Fisher there were many contributors to statistical theory. Subsequent advances in methodology were mainly refinements and elaborations. Thus, when nursing research began to expand in the 1950s, statistical methodology was fully developed and became an important influence on the quantitative orientation of nursing studies. Moreover, the work of the social scientists Thorndike, Thurstone, Likert, and Guttman in developing methodology for sociological and psychological research, primarily in defining, scaling, and quantifying qualitative variables, was becoming widely known by 1950 and also exerted an influence on nursing studies.

Statistical methodology has thus evolved from descriptive analysis of large bodies of data to explanatory analysis of data gathered in tightly controlled experimental studies. The methodology is utilized in all forms of research in which the data are quantitative. Indeed, statistics has become closely intertwined with research methodology. To some, research methodology and statistical methodology are synonymous.

The Role of Statistical Methodology in Nursing Research

Quantitative research is an orderly and systematic approach for collecting and analyzing data. The term "rigor" is applied to quantitative research, meaning that it will be conducted according to a set of prescribed rules that promote objectivity, precision, and correctness. The use of statistical methods helps achieve rigor in research.

Quantification and statistical methodology permeate phases of the quantitative research process. Statistical methods are especially important in the following phases:

- Describing the conceptual and theoretical framework;
- Stating hypotheses;
- Delineating study variables and determining how to measure them;

- Selecting the study subjects; and
- Analyzing the data.

Conceptual Framework

Ever since Rogers (1970) emphasized the importance of nursing theories to the creation of a scientific basis for nursing, nursing research has placed considerable emphasis on conceptual frameworks and theories as foundations of any research effort (Fitzpatrick & Whall, 1983). As Cohen and Nagel have stated (1934, p. 399), "theories have been successful in coordinating vast domains of phenomena, and fertile in making discoveries of the most important kind."

Many examples can be found in the nursing research literature of the use of theoretical and conceptual frameworks. In a study of the compliance of hypertensive patients with the prescribed treatment regimen, for example, Fishbein's *theory of reasoned action* was used to delineate study hypotheses and variables (Miller, Wikoff, & Hiatt, 1992). This theory clarified the relationships among the study variables and suggested how they should be measured.

Conceptual frameworks often lay the groundwork for the statistical aspects of quantitative research. They can operationally define the variables in quantitative terms. They can postulate a relationship among variables that identifies the statistical technique to be used in evaluating the relationship. And, in turn, statistics can be benefit the formulation of frameworks. As stated by Kaplan (1964, p. 51), "The statistical approach in general has the merit of providing warrant for a conceptualization which may have heuristic value even though it does not wholly solve the scientific problem to which it is addressed."

Hypotheses

Defined simply as a statement of the relationship among the phenomena being studied, hypothesis are derived from the conceptual framework. They serve to organize and guide the research. The culmination of many quantitative studies is the statistical test of the hypotheses that have been stated.

Statistical hypothesis-testing is a major use of statistical methodology in quantitative nursing research, particularly in studies that experimentally test the effects of interventions. Commonly, the underlying model in such tests is the general linear hypothesis, simply stated as $y = f(x)$, in which the intervention is x and the effect (outcome) is y, both measured quantitatively. Many statistical techniques exist to test hypotheses, and quantitative research makes extensive use of them as even a superficial perusal of the nursing research literature will reveal.

Study Variables

Quantitative research deals with quantified variables; that is, with scales of measurement that provide quantified values. Statistical methodology is very useful in assessing the validity and reliability of measures of quantified variables. It is also useful in evaluating and improving the sensitivity of measures. As Stewart and Archbold (1992) have stated, a measure may be valid and reliable, but it is useless if its scale is unresponsive to clinically significant changes in the study subjects.

Researchers frequently use measures of variables for their research that have been developed by others rather than invent new ones. Statistical techniques can be very helpful in selecting and utilizing existing measures. An example of this is provided by Strauss (1988), who studied the variable "information-seeking behavior" of hospitalized surgical patients. The measure used was developed by statistically evaluating the reliability and validity of two existing measures and revising the coding and scoring methods.

Selecting Study Subjects

Statistical techniques play an important role in the determination of the *method* of selecting a *sample* of study subjects and the *size* of the sample. However, the techniques apply only if the sample is *randomly* and not *purposively* selected, as study subjects often are in nursing studies. Various methods exist for drawing random samples. These range from the aptly named simple, unrestricted samples, in which each member of the population from which the sample is drawn has an equal chance of being selected for the study, to complex multi-stage samples involving repeated random sampling from various layers or strata of the population to arrive at the sample of study subjects as was done in a study of nursing home patients (Algase, 1992).

The question of how large a sample should be depends on the variability of the measure among the members of the population as well as how much error the researcher is willing to tolerate in drawing inferences from the sample data. The impact of variability is obvious.

The smaller the variability of the measure, the smaller is the error for a given sample size; if there were no variability, a sample of one would be adequate. Sample size can also be reduced if a larger error can be tolerated in the value of the measure being studied.

While it is desirable to minimize sample size in order to limit research costs, small samples are not necessarily the best samples. Small samples cannot provide the rich descriptive information of large samples. Moreover, in testing hypotheses concerning *effects* of interventions, the *power* of the test to detect statistically significant differences among comparison groups decreases as sample size decreases. But power is not the ultimate criterion of quality of the quantitative research design. A poorly designed and executed study is likely to produce spurious results, no matter how large the sample.

Analyzing Data

Statistical methodology plays its largest role in quantitative research in data analysis, the aim of which is "to provide insight by means of numbers" (Moore, 1985, p. *vi*). Statistical analysis of research data is essentially an inferential process of drawing statistical conclusions from the data. Research data are sample data, and the aim of the analysis is to infer them to a larger population.

Textbooks on statistical methods, as well as many nursing research textbooks, devote more space to data analysis than to any other topic. Suffice to say that analytical techniques can be arranged into three categories, according to whether the data to which they are applied are univariable, bivariable, or multivariable. Univariable data are data on a single variable and the analysis focuses on its behavior. The role of statistical methodology in univariable analysis consists of computing summary measures—averages, relative frequencies, variances, etc.—and determining sampling errors of the measures in order to infer population estimates of the variable. For example: "In 1988, 7.6 percent of all registered nurses were from racial/ethnic minority backgrounds" (Moses, 1990, p. 14).

The analysis of bivariable data focuses on the *relationship* between two variables. When a substantively meaningful relationship between two variables is hypothesized, as in evaluating the effects on patients of clinical interventions, one variable is said to be dependent on the other, which is called the independent variable. The main purpose of the study is to infer the hypothesized *relationship* to a larger population rather than inferring the values of measures of individual variables. Statistical techniques of correlation analysis, one-way analysis of variance, and simple regression analysis are used to evaluate bivariable relationships.

As nursing research has advanced and hypotheses have become more complex, the use of statistical techniques to analyze multivariable data has become commonplace. The relationship among a single dependent variable and multiple independent variables can be evaluated by such techniques as multiple regression and two-way analysis of variance. In the more complex case of multiple dependent as well as multiple independent variables, the analytical techniques of *multivariate* analysis, such as multivariate analysis of variance and discriminant analysis, can be applied (Dillon & Goldstein, 1984). Computers have made even the most sophisticated techniques relatively quick and easy to use.

Uses and Limits of Quantitative Research

Uses and Advantages

There is little doubt that quantitative research using statistical methodology has been helpful in advancing nursing as a scientific discipline. It has been especially useful in studies that aim to solve a problem or to evaluate those aspects of nursing that can be measured.

There are many advantages to using quantification in nursing research. There are many tools of statistical analysis available that can be applied to almost any conceivable research topic. The results of quantitative studies look impressive, with lots of neatly arranged numbers in statistical tables and mathematical formulas to back up the analysis and give the study a certain mathematical elegance. The findings of quantitative studies are generally easy to communicate because numbers are a universal language. Results of quantitative studies on similar topics can be conveniently synthesized, thus facilitating the accumulation of knowledge.

Many write-ups of nursing studies consist almost entirely of statistical description and analysis. Nurse researchers appear to be very comfortable using quantitative research methodology. Nursing studies utilize the full range of statistical techniques including some that are rarely applied in other fields of research. Reports of nursing studies are steeped in the language of statistical methodology, especially when a co-author is a statistician.

As the trend in the use of quantitative research in nursing appears to be upward, the forecast for the 21st century is for continued and increasing usage. The upward trend will be facilitated by further advances in computerization, further development of statistical techniques, particularly for multivariable analysis, and the creation of large-scale databases into which nurse researchers can tap. The future is indeed rosy for quantitative research, but a few cautions are in order to avoid the pitfalls of "over-quantification."

Limitations and Cautions

There is a danger that overreliance on quantification and statistical analysis in nursing research can have adverse consequences. As to quantification, reducing everything to numbers not only may result in data that has little real-world reality, but may drain all descriptive richness from the phenomenon being studied. For example, operationally defining nursing care as the amount of time nurses spend on the nursing unit removes the qualitative depth with which care-giving can be described. Such a definition may be sufficient for a management study, but is grossly inadequate for a clinical study that is evaluating the impact of nursing interventions on recipients of care.

Overreliance on statistical analysis has led to misuses and overuses of inferential statistics, particularly tests of significance. The use of these tests has to meet certain requirements and assumptions that are frequently ignored. It seems that some researchers look to the techniques to add a scientific gloss to the findings. Why use methodology when a straightforward interpretation of the study results, minus the statistical tests, will not only avoid misuse, but will concentrate the researcher's attention on the real meaning of the data? The danger is that fascination with methodology diverts attention from substance to process.

Nurse researchers should take care not to become more like statisticians than researchers. Statistical methodology includes not one, but several full-time occupations and specialties: design, measurement, sampling, and analysis. Nurse researchers do not have to be experts in all methodological fields; they should call upon consultants as needed. What will be helpful to nurse researchers in the future is a good knowledge of how statistical methodology can assist research, the limits of this methodology, and how statistical reasoning is applied to the interpretation of research data.

The remainder of this part of the book is organized as follows. The next chapter will discuss qualitative research, which is at the other end of the research methodology spectrum. Successive chapters will contain discussions of selected topics primarily within the area of quantitative research, beginning with clinical trials. Some topics addressed in this chapter, such as uses and misuses of statistical tests of significance, will reappear for further discussion. An underlying theme of all chapters of this book is preparation for nursing research in the future.

Chapter 5

Qualitative Research

What is Qualitative Research?

The term "qualitative research" is confusing. To some it connotes research on the "quality of care" or some other "qualitative" issue. Prior to the burgeoning interest in qualitative research, the term "qualitative" was almost always used in quantitative research to denote a particular kind of variable, one in which the scale of measurement is expressed qualitatively rather than quantitatively, as was discussed in the last chapter.

If qualitative research does not mean research on quality of care or research that uses qualitative scales, what does it mean? It is difficult to find a simple definition. Qualitative researchers do not always agree on a definition. Some regard it as a philosophical approach to research and not as a methodology. Where most do seem to agree is that qualitative research avoids quantification.

Qualitative research can be defined as *research without measurement*. Instead of measuring variables, qualitative researchers make narrative recordings of the phenomena they are studying using interviews and direct observation. This material can be in the form of verbatim or short-hand text, or it can be reduced to codes. It can even be in raw form as in audio or video recordings. It is probably accurate to describe the methodology of qualitative research as loosely structured and free-flowing. The processes of data gathering, analysis, and interpretation are closely linked in qualitative research and may be carried out simultaneously (Patton, 1990).

According to Strauss (1987), a major distinction between qualitative and quantitative research is that the former focuses on situational and structural contexts, whereas the latter focuses on relationships among quantified variables. Since qualitative research deemphasizes the measurement of variables, the data are stronger on context, but weaker on cross-comparisons.

Characteristics of Qualitative Research

It is perhaps easiest to explain what qualitative research is by discussing some of its characteristics.

The Practice of Nursing is Congenial to Qualitative Research

Qualitative research applications in nursing originated in the 1960s at the same time that the term *qualitative research* first appeared in the social science research literature. Previously, nursing research had consisted of descriptive studies of the role of the nurse and industrial engineering studies of nursing efficiency. In the early 1960s social scientists became involved in nursing research, and nursing studies began to be increasingly based on models and theories of human behavior. The emphasis on social interactions and contextual and situational phenomena stimulated a demand for research methods that would holistically capture the richness of the experiences of nurses and patients that quantitative research could only superficially address.

Qualitative Research is Strongly Linked to the Social and Behavioral Sciences

Qualitative research, originating in the social and behavioral sciences, has been almost entirely applied to these discipline areas, especially sociology and anthropology. Terms used to describe qualitative methodologies such as phenomenology, ethnography, and grounded theory have a strong social science flavor. Much of the qualitative research conducted in nursing has employed theoretical perspectives, philosophies, and terminology from the social and behavioral sciences. By contrast, quantitative research is discipline-free and can be applied to virtually any subject matter including, of course, the social and behavioral sciences.

The Data of Qualitative Research are Rich in Detail

Data collection techniques used in qualitative research include participant observations, interviews, questionnaires, and anecdotal recordings. Its open-ended structure permits freer responses than do the closed-end instruments of quantitative research. The technique of *content analysis*, which is basically an analytical method, can be used in qualitative research to gather data on secondary material such as historical records. The *case study* method provides a detailed collection of narrative, anecdotal data on a small set of subjects, such as a single individual or group. While data from these studies are rich in detail, they have limited generalizability.

In quantitative research the data are typically less detailed. They are reduced, summarized, and episodic, but the larger number of subjects sampled and a research design that focuses on relationships among variables facilitates generalization of findings. Generalizing results from a qualitative study is not usually a prime objective, however. The intent is an improved understanding of human behavior and relationships through an in-depth examination of real-life experiences.

Qualitative Research is Process Oriented

Essentially, qualitative research attempts to answer questions of *process*—"How does something happen?"—whereas quantitative studies focus on *outcomes*—"What happens if....?" Qualitative studies usually have a longer-range objective than do quantitative studies: they are intended to generate explanatory theories rather than test products or solve problems (Denzin & Lincoln, 1994).

Data Collection and Data Analysis are Intertwined in Qualitative Research

In contrast to quantitative research, where the data collection and analysis processes are compartmentalized and rigidly standardized in order to enhance objectivity, qualitative methods allow a subjective approach to data. Qualitative researchers may analyze the data as they are collected, thus playing a direct role in both data collection and analysis. Data collection and analysis in quantitative research leave little room for interpretive creativity until after the data have been processed.

There are Concerns About the "Scientific" Worth of Qualitative Research

Qualitative studies are criticized by quantitative researchers as being "soft" research, lacking in rigor and scientific objectivity (Clarke, 1992). The unstructured, free-flowing, and somewhat subjective aspects of qualitative methods are unfavorably compared to the mathematical "purity" and objectivity of quantitative techniques. The limitations of qualitative research in making generalizations of data to a larger population, particularly about causal relationships, is considered a major limitation. Needless to say, some of these criticisms arise from a misunderstanding of the goals of qualitative studies.

Qualitative Research is Compatible with Quantitative Research

Qualitative research is not a substitute for quantitative research; and vice versa. It is not an "either/or" situation. For most research purposes one methodology cannot be substituted for the other. Although the two types of research use different approaches and techniques to collect and analyze different kinds of data, they are not incompatible, but can be complementary in carrying out nursing research that requires diversified approaches (Jicks, 1979; Murphy, 1989). Research combining qualitative and quantitative approaches can use the former to good advantage in the early exploratory phase of the study, in the interpretative stage, and in theory development. A combined approach, called *triangulation,* can enhance comprehensiveness of findings and provide data to cross-validate conclusions (Goodwin & Goodwin, 1984).

Qualitative Research is a Strategy for Research, not a "Sealed in Concrete" Methodology

The aims of qualitative research methodology are to provide a summary and synthesis of a researcher's experience of the informant's reality. It can be viewed as a set of purposeful strategies rather than hard and fast methodological rules (Marshall & Rossman, 1989). It is not cook-book research, but, rather, highly individualistic and dependent on the particular investigatory style of the researcher.

Qualitative Research Uses Inductive Reasoning

Qualitative researchers claim that they use the *inductive* method, while quantitative research uses the *deductive* method. As defined by Cohen and Nagel in their classic book on logic and scientific method (1934), induction is "the process of generalization, the passage from a statement true of some observed instances to a statement true of all possible instances of a certain class." Conversely, the deductive method begins with general propositions (theories, hypotheses) and evaluates their application to real-life instances.

In other words, induction goes from the particular to the general (observations to theories) whereas deduction goes from the general to the particular (theories to observations). However, this distinction is not entirely accurate when used to differentiate qualitative from quantitative research. Although it is true that much qualitative research begins with observation of specific experiences and aims at generating broadly applicable propositions about human behavior, the objective of many quantitative studies is, also, to produce theories. The hypotheses of many quantitative studies are tentative and speculative. The expectation is that their confirmation or refutation of the collected data will contribute to theory development.

The Evolution of Qualitative Research

Whereas early examples of the philosophy and procedures of qualitative research can be found in the studies of social anthropologists such as the Lynds (1929), Benedict (1934), and Mead (1939), the term "qualitative research", designating a completely distinct and comprehensive methodological approach to research, is of recent origin. Interestingly, one of the earliest uses of the term can be found in the nursing journal, *Nursing Research*, used by researchers who had undertaken a study of death and dying (Glaser & Strauss, 1966). Textbooks on general applications of the methodology began to appear in the 1970s followed by nursing applications in the 1980s (Leininger, 1985; Munhall & Oiler, 1986).

Unlike the evolution of quantitative methodology, in which there has been a steady course of elaborations and refinements of earlier techniques, progress in qualitative methodology has not been as smooth. In fact, it is difficult to discern the significant trends in this methodology since it first appeared on the nursing scene some 30 years ago.

Qualitative research methodology, as has been stated, originated in the social sciences, in the field of cultural anthropology. Long before qualitative research methods were used to study health problems, social science theories and models had begun to have an influence on the delivery of health care. Flexner (1925), in his study of medical education, described the interrelationships between the physical and social sciences in the optimal care of the patient. MacIver (1937) and Lynd (1939) discussed how the social sciences could address problems of health and illness. It is interesting to note that the book entitled *Social Science in Medicine* (Simmons & Wolff, 1954), was published a year prior to the initiation of the federal government's program of support for nursing research in 1955.

Following on the heels of Simmons and Wolff was the publication in 1960 of Macgregor's *Social Science in Nursing* which discussed the implications of the social sciences for nursing care. Describing the numerous social, psychological, and cultural factors that play important roles in a person's health status, she urged the inclusion of the principles and methodologies of the social sciences in nursing education and research. Macgregor also explained the benefits of a qualitative approach in nursing research. She used the term qualitative research to describe anthropological research in which the "task is not so much that of asking questions, as discovering what *kinds* of questions to ask." According to Macgregor, the objective of qualitative research is not to aggregate large quantities of measurements of fragmented variables, but, rather, to uncover recurring patterns of behavior.

Macgregor's book helped to introduce more social and behavioral science content into the nursing curriculum. But her promotion of qualitative methodology did not have an immediate impact on nursing research, although nursing studies began to make more use of theories and models from the social and behavioral sciences. The prevailing methodology in these studies, as in social science research in general, was quantitative, meaning that the main attributes of the methodology included the following: measurement, objective data collection, assessment of validity and reliability, statistical analysis of data, use of statistical inference to generalize findings, and replication of studies using identical designs.

The Strauss study (1963) of dying patients, one of the first nursing studies to use qualitative methodology, was conducted shortly after the publication of *Social Science in Nursing* (Glaser & Strauss, 1965). Glaser and Strauss (1967) then published a lengthy discussion of a qualitative research technique which they called *grounded theory*. There followed an acceleration of interest in qualitative methodology, and today many examples can be found of the uses of this and other qualitative research methodology in nursing research (Vehvilainer-Julikunen, 1992).

Applications in Nursing Research

Although quantitative methodology still dominates nursing research, including studies with a social or behavioral science orientation, qualitative approaches have received increased attention, especially in the past 10 years due, to the following factors:

An Increase in the Number of Nurses Educated in the Social and Behavioral Sciences

The number of nurses obtaining graduate education increased after passage of the federal government's Nurse Traineeship Program (1956) and the Nurse Training Act (1964). The curricula included courses in the social and behavioral sciences, and theses and dissertations containing sociological, psychological, and anthropological content began to apply qualitative methods such as grounded theory, phenomenology, and ethnography (Strauss & Corbin, 1990; Wondoloski, 1991).

Development of Models and Theories Has Increased

An active period of model and theory development in nursing began in the 1970s as a natural off-shoot of the expanded research initiative. This development has served to stimulate qualitative research, since the primary objective of many qualitative studies is theory development.

Expansion of the Literature on Nursing Research

In the past twenty years, the number of journal articles and books on qualitative research has increased considerably. Workshops and conferences have been held on qualitative methods. There are now organizations of qualitative researchers. Increased communication has stimulated applications of the methodology to nursing topics.

Expansion of Nursing Research into a Variety of Areas of Human Behavior has led to Increased Reliance on Qualitative Data and Methods to Analyze Them

Nursing draws from many different areas of human knowledge, including the physical and biological sciences as well as the social and behavioral sciences. The variety of nursing research content has stimulated the use of qualitative methods, as the following titles of actual studies indicate:

- Hospitalization of severely burned school-aged children;
- Post-operative pain in preschool children;
- Patients on a cancer unit;
- Weaning patterns of first-time mothers;
- Touching behaviors of intensive care nurses;
- Behaviors of preschoolers in intensive care;
- The human experience of miscarriage;
- Transitions over the life cycle;
- Anxieties and concerns of acutely ill patients;
- Transformation of woman to mother;
- Restlessness;
- Suicidal behavior;
- The role of men in family planning clinics;
- Reactions of elderly persons to entry to nursing homes; and
- Living with persons undergoing chemotherapy.

These titles show topics that range over a wide spectrum of subjects and problems with a strong sociological or psychological flavor. Children's issue loom large in these studies as do problems pertaining to women's role in society.

A down-to-earth quality is inherent in these projects. They are directed towards relevant, timely, and important problems. Although the nursing content of some may be difficult to discern from the titles, the potential usefulness of the studies to the practice of nursing is, in each case, arguably quite high. In fact, if a list of topics were to be randomly selected from recently published quantitative studies in nursing, it is likely that they would not be consistently focused on issues having as practical implications for nursing practice as do these qualitative studies.

Because qualitative research applications to nursing are of recent origin, it is difficult to assess the status of dissemination and utilization of study findings. Review of the topics of completed research does show that they address areas of importance to nursing: pregnancy, family planning, anxiety about hospitalization, aging, dying, and responses to institutionalization. To a large extent these findings are descriptive rather than explanatory or evaluative. It is much simpler to use the findings of quantitative research that concludes that method A reduced bedsores in patients by 50% as compared to method B than to provide a large amount of narrative data that describes the *process* of bedsores. However, the wealth of descriptive data may be valuable in generating a *theory* of bedsores that has the potential for providing a more substantial and longer lasting solution to the problem than does the quantitative study.

Limitations and Strengths of Qualitative and Quantitative Research

Any discussion of the limitations and strengths of qualitative and quantitative research must start with a critique of the categorization itself. Dichotomizing research methodology this way may not be constructive. Among the consequences is an adversarial posture among researchers who champion one approach or the other. This has led to claims that "my method is better than yours," implying that the different approaches are interchangeable depending on the background and inclination of the researcher.

The Concepts of Quality and Quantity

Apropos of what can be described as the rivalry between qualitative and quantitative researchers, Kaplan (1964, p. 206) discusses the mystique surrounding the words "quality" and "quantity." The mystique of quality is more pernicious in its effect because, according to Kaplan, advocates view numbers with great distaste, believing that their use is "a kind of black magic, effective only for evil ends, and seducing us into giving up our souls for what, after all is nothing but dross." On the other hand, the mystique of quantity maintains that if you cannot get something down to numbers that can be objectively measured, it is not worth pursuing. This attitude holds that measurement is a necessary condition for scientific progress.

The fact is that quality and quantity are not antithetical concepts, but are quite compatible. As Kaplan (1964, p. 207) so aptly puts it, "quantities are of qualities and a measured quality *has* just the magnitude expressed in its measure."

The term quality embraces a variety of concepts—attribute, characteristic, property, class, kind, grade, distinction, trait, capacity, virtue—to list only the more common ones. In the terminology of statistical methodology a quality is labeled a variable if, as is true of most if not all conceivable qualities, it contains a scale of categories or gradations that can be described verbally or in numbers. Thus, the quality "color" can be verbally described as green or red, or in numbers as the wavelength of the color as measured by an electronic apparatus. Similarly, the quality "weight" can be described as heavy or light, or in numbers obtained by applying a mechanical or electronic apparatus.

Numbers can also be generated for a quality even if it does not have a numerical scale or if appropriate apparatus does not exist (Bryman, 1988). The qualitative distinctions of the attribute compose the scale, for example, red, green, orange (nominal ungraded scale), or small, medium, large (ordinal graded scale). When these scales are used in research, quantities are obtained by counting the number of study subjects having each distinction of the scale, which is essentially a form of binary measurement; i.e., the subject has the attribute or does not have the attribute.

Purposes of Qualitative and Quantitative Research

What value is there in labeling research as qualitative or quantitative? A more useful classification might well be according to purpose and not whether measurement is used or not. The short-term purpose of many qualitative studies seems to be to compile in-depth narrative descriptions of the complexities of human behavior, while the long-range purpose is to use these data in theory development. Of course, some quantitative studies have these same purposes.

An important characteristic of qualitative methodology is that it puts the researcher squarely into the data collection and analysis phases of the study. The qualitative researcher has considerable flexibility in pursuing promising new areas of investigation by changing the course spelled out in the original research plan. However, unless the specific purpose is clearly spelled out in advance, this flexibility may make it difficult to see where the research is heading. Labeling research of this kind as *exploratory* accurately describes its purpose while not denigrating its significance.

Quantitative research is purposeful: it is designed to test, compare, trouble-shoot, discover causes, predict. Some of these purposes, notably testing and trouble-shooting, are inappropriate for qualitative research because verbal description alone cannot provide the appropriate needed data. The purposes of much quantitative research can be subsumed under the heading of *evaluation*, which has been defined as an effort to enhance human effectiveness through systematic, data-based inquiry (Patton, 1990).

As opposed to the greater flexibility offered by qualitative research, there are considerably more constraints on the quantitative researcher in carrying out evaluation studies. Many of the specifications of the design of the research—hypotheses, samples, measuring instruments, and analytical techniques—are determined prior to data collection and cannot be significantly changed during the study without threatening its validity. The data collection and analysis phases of an evaluation study should be independent and compartmentalized. The study must be administered and documented so that it can be replicated. Objectivity is paramount. And, unlike qualitative research in which the researcher can take some liberties with various aspects of the research design, the quantitative researcher is strictly bound by the protocol.

Limitations of Qualitative Research

Some advocates of qualitative research have a tendency to exaggerate its virtues, even claiming that it is superior to quantitative research. There are certainly good things to be said about the qualitative approach, but its limitations must also be recognized. It is useful to restate some of these limitations. Understanding them helps to make better use of the methodology and improve utilization of findings.

Limited Applications

A major purpose of qualitative research is to explore an issue in great detail and depth. It cannot be used to test an hypothesis, investigate causal relationships, or make predictions, because these purposes require a controlled and systematic design in which numerical data are collected from comparison groups. One important aim of qualitative research is theory development, but any theory is in its nature speculative and provisional and must be tested in controlled studies to be widely accepted.

Limited Generalizability of Findings

Qualitative research gathers a great wealth of data from a very small sample, sometimes even a sample of one subject. Moreover, study subjects are not selected from a larger population according to the rules of random sampling. In fact, qualitative researchers advocate the use of purposive sampling to obtain the most appropriate subjects. The virtue of random sampling is that it controls for *biased* selection of study subjects. Without it the researcher may select study subjects because they are cooperative or convenient. Selected purposively, the sample could very easily contain atypical representatives of the population and lead to spurious inferences. Random sampling not only leaves the selection of subjects to chance, but also makes it possible to compute measures of sampling error for the study findings when they are generalized. These measures are necessary to the determination of the statistical significance of the data.

Qualitative Data are Soft

Although narrative data may be quite expressive and descriptive and provide a richness that numerical data lack, they can also be ambiguous and imprecise. This can lead to misunderstanding and disagreement. In clinical situations reliance on nonquantitative data would be unacceptable. To say that a patient's blood pressure is "high" is a weak and imprecise statement compared to stating that the patient's blood pressure is 250/110. Even in nonclinical situations, as Kaplan (1964) remarks, categories such as senior citizen, well-to-do, or feeble-minded, are more difficult, if not impossible, to put to scientific use than the corresponding quantitative specifications of age, income, or intelligence. But quantification is not without its limitations. In complex situations of social interaction, measurement may only provide a shallow, one-sided, fragmented, and even misleading description of the real world.

What is the Research Design?

Quantitative research uses formal and well-structured designs. The term "experiment" connotes a clearly defined structure and process for conducting research. So do terms such as "survey," "*ex post facto* design," and "control group." The language of quantitative research is relatively easy to communicate to others. This is not so for qualitative research. Terms such as "ethnography," "phenomenology," "hermeneutics," and "grounded theory" are not familiar to the general research community. It is not entirely clear that these are methodological terms, and if they are, what specifically are the characteristics of the methodology that bear these labels? Qualitative researchers shy away from standardization (although not from systemization), claiming that each research project must have its own special, customized sequence of steps—the researcher follows where the data lead (Strauss, 1987). However, if a research project is to maximally contribute to the advancement of a nursing science, it must have a rational and objective process, capable of being understood, repeated, and verified by others.

Analytical Techniques are Limited

Many qualitative studies use *content analysis* as their analytical method. The raw verbal data are arranged into a cognitive or semantic schemata consisting of categories that have some relationship to each other and some degree of mutual exclusiveness. How these are utilized in theory development, or if not theory, in general conclusions, is not exactly clear. The analytical approach is only understood from the verbal description provided in the report of each individual research project.

In contrast, the analysis stage of quantitative research is one of its strengths. The use of measurement makes possible the application of a well-developed, objective, and highly effective set of techniques known as statistical methodology. These techniques are available for every step in the research process: statement of hypotheses, sampling of the population, specification of the variables under study and instruments to measure them, aggregation, reduction, and summarization of data, assessment of sampling error, determination of statistical significance of data findings, and evaluation of data reliability and validity. The powerful techniques of statistical methodology have been made even more powerful by the computer. Although some computer software, such as *Ethnograph* and *Qualpro*, is available for analyzing verbal text for qualitative research, the major contribution of computer technology lies in its superb handling of numerical data.

Costs are High

It would be interesting to do a comparative cost-benefit analysis of qualitative and quantitative research projects, especially for projects in which the research content and purpose are similar. Without the data from such an analysis it might be tempting to conclude that the qualitative approach is the more expensive type of research because of the collection of large amounts of narrative data. Collecting data through field observation and open-ended interviews, especially when a senior researcher is involved, can be time-consuming and costly.

By contrast, questionnaires, structured interviews, and the use of certain measuring instruments provide comparatively cheap techniques for gathering numerical data from large samples of study subjects in a short time. However, clinical research can also be very expensive when it employs complex physiological measurements and subjects are repeatedly evaluated.

For both methods costs can be reduced by using secondary data sources such as records, transcripts, newspapers, films, and data collected in other studies, including databases that are constructed from large scale record-keeping systems and files such as Medicare. Data collection can be made more efficient and effective through the use of indirect measures that are not literal constructs of the variable being measured. Projective techniques are good examples of indirect measures. The ultimate consideration must be the benefits achieved with the method used. There is little value in employing an expensive research design or complicated data-gathering instruments if they produce trivia.

Difficult to Replicate

It is difficult to replicate qualitative studies because of lack of standardization of various elements of the research design as well as their subjective style. Nevertheless, it is desirable to accumulate the results of replicated qualitative studies when possible. Replication of studies and accumulation of results are essential to the construction of a scientific body of knowledge. The findings of a study, particularly in clinical nursing where they could directly affect people's health, must be confirmed by other studies before implementation.

Difficult to Evaluate

A common criticism of qualitative research is that it avoids the issues of reliability and validity, concepts that are usually applied to the data collection (measurement) phase of a study, although applicable to other phases too: sample, analytical method, interpretation. They are omitted from consideration in qualitative research because it is believed that they are only applicable to quantitative research.

Other criteria for evaluating qualitative research have been put forward: substance, clarity, integration, conceptual dimension, and interpretive soundness (Parse, Coyne, & Smith, 1985). These criteria seem to be more applicable to the report-writing stage of research than to methodology. The concepts of reliability and validity, as well as other criteria usually applied to quantitative research, such as relevance, sensitivity, completeness, and generality of findings *are* applicable to qualitative studies. How else can research findings be evaluated? Thus, for example, if a researcher using a qualitative approach concludes that teenage girls who avoid prenatal care have had little prior experience with any kind of health care, would other researchers independently pursuing this topic arrive at the same conclusion? How extensively can the findings of this study be generalized, considering that it was done in a single, purposively chosen health center and involved only a small number of subjects? Until these and similar questions can be answered, qualitative research findings will have limited usefulness.

Future Role of Qualitative Research in Nursing

The discussion of the limitations of qualitative research was not intended to denigrate its usefulness as an approach to conducting a nursing study. Understanding these limitations can only result in a more realistic and accurate assessment of its potential contributions to future research.

Projecting the future role of the qualitative approach in nursing research should begin with an understanding of its strengths. Qualitative research refers to the methods and techniques of observing, recording, analyzing, and interpreting the attributes, patterns, linkages, directionality, and meanings of specific properties of the phenomena under investigation (Leininger, 1985). The phenomena studied are primarily human interactions in social settings. They are studied holistically, in depth, and with an attempt to describe the "lived experience" in which these phenomena occur. In short, the data of qualitative research are imbued with realism.

Comparatively speaking, qualitative research is stronger on description and weaker on analysis, whereas quantitative research is weaker on description and stronger on analysis. The verbal description of qualitative studies can better capture the contextual characteristics of the phenomena under study holistically, realistically, and dynamically than can quantitative studies, which examine phenomena discretely, summarily, and abstractly. Consider the following difference in the way phenomena are described.

Qualitative: The patient is an older, feeble male who needs assistance with feeding and bathing. Although not completely bedridden, he spends almost no time out of bed, usually sitting in a chair while his bed is being made. His hypotension makes him lightheaded at times. He is cooperative and obliging, and apologizes each time he has to use the call bell for assistance. He is not particularly interested in reading or in watching television and spends much time staring into space. He enjoys talking to people, especially about his experiences as a longshoreman after he graduated from high school. He rarely mentions his health problem, chronic obstructive pulmonary disease, which he attributes to heavy smoking as a youth. He is not optimistic about being cured of this problem, but is hoping he will make sufficient recovery to become ambulatory again and be able to return home.

Quantitative: Patient M, 74 years of age, Education 12 yrs, DRG 88, 4 yrs duration, ADL 3.3, Mental Status 1.8, BP 90/56.

It is obvious that the qualitative data provide a richer and denser description of the patient and his condition, but they are not readily amenable to analysis and interpretation. The quantitative data are fragmented, sparse, and sharply focused, but can be subjected to analysis by a wide array of statistical methods.

It is immediately obvious that the two sets of data can and should be used to complement and supplement each other. Commentaries on the uses to which qualitative research can be put call this integration of approaches "triangulation" (Knafl & Breitmayer, 1991). The qualitative method can be useful in the exploratory phases of a triangulated approach to investigate in depth the background and context of the research problem. It can also be profitably applied to gather data when instruments to measure quantitative variables are unavailable. The qualitative approach can also be helpful in the end stages of a research project to obtain a richer understanding of the meaning of the data and to give the research report a realistic and worldly flavor (Tilden, Nelson, & May, 1990).

An especially fruitful area for the application of qualitative methodology in future nursing studies is health promotion and disease prevention (HPDP). First, it is important because nurses can play a key role in carrying out HPDP efforts. Second, HPDP accomplishments depend on a sound understanding of the behavioral aspects involved, including knowledge of the lifestyle changes necessary to reduce health risks. Third, the National Institutes of Health are placing much emphasis on achieving the HPDP goals of the U.S. Department of Health and Human Services *Healthy People 2000* (1991). Research proposals that directly address these goals will receive extra consideration in the determination of their priority scores for funding support.

To close this chapter, some nursing research topics that might lend themselves to the qualitative approach include:

- Eating behaviors of obese persons;
- Characteristics of teen-age mothers;
- Mothers of extremely low birth-weight infants;
- Smoking and excessive alcohol consumption;
- Violent behavior and relationship to other factors;
- Impact of Alzheimer's disease on family members;
- Homelessness and health status;
- Context of the quality of nursing care;
- Reasons for avoidance of prenatal care;
- Motivating people towards healthier lifestyles;
- Depression in different age groups; and
- Health education content of nursing care in hospitals.

Chapter 6

Clinical Trials

Overview

The clinical trial as a type of research design stands in sharp contrast to qualitative research. Whereas qualitative research observes human behavior as "life as being lived," a clinical trial uses the *experimental design* as its model. In a clinical trial the researcher introduces an intervention in a clinical environment to evaluate its effects on human study subjects.

A clinical trial is among the most quantitative of all research approaches (Mason, Gunst & Hess, 1989). The effects of interventions are measured as precisely as possible and high-powered statistical techniques are employed to evaluate them against a control (Friedman, Furberg, & DeMets, 1984). Interventions in clinical trials can include prophylactic, diagnostic, or therapeutic agents, frequently pharmaceuticals. Clinical trials also evaluate medical devices, procedures, techniques, and regimens (Easterbrook, 1992; National Institutes of Health, 1975).

Clinical trials are, thus, a form of evaluation research. They are intended to produce results that have immediate, clinical applications. Qualitative research and other forms of basic research are far removed from the short-range, practical aims of clinical trials.

Humans are the research subjects in clinical trials, although animals may be used in the early stages of the testing of drugs and other therapies. Effects of interventions in clinical trials are often measured by physiologic variables, employing quantitative scales. Functional capabilities of people in the activities of daily living (ADL), measured by qualitative scales are also frequently used to measure effects (outcomes) of interventions.

A key feature of clinical trials is the control group, which serves as the basis of comparison of the effects that occur in the group receiving the intervention, known as the treatment, test, intervention, or experimental group. Members of the control group either do not receive the intervention or else receive a different version or level of the intervention. The control group should be comparable to the treatment group; the two groups should be balanced in terms of variables that could significantly affect the impact of the intervention, for example, age, because older people react differently to drugs and to other interventions than do younger people.

In order for statistical techniques to be validly applied to data, subjects must be assigned to the treatment or control group by chance, through a random process. Although randomization does not insure perfect equivalence of the groups in relation to the multitude of variables present in human subjects (especially in small samples), it theoretically should provide as reasonably balanced groups as possible and, in any case, it prevents the biases that can occur by deliberately assigning someone to a treatment group because the researcher believes that a good outcome will result. Techniques such as *covariance analysis*, in which baseline measurements are taken before any interventions are introduced, often are used to further improve comparability of treatment and control groups.

Clinical trials have not been widely used in research designs for nursing studies. Deterrents to its use are the high costs and technical difficulties associated with the conduct of such rigorously controlled studies (Abdellah, 1990). Some researchers criticize clinical trials as being too closely tied to the medical model and not without reason. In the future, though, it can be expected that greater use will be made of clinical trials to evaluate the different nursing interventions, regimens, tools, and techniques that have evolved over the past 50 years.

What are Clinical Trials?

The randomized clinical trial, or RCT for short, has been called the "gold standard" for the design of studies to evaluate the effectiveness of medical interventions (Rabeneck, Viscoli & Horwitz, 1992). As has been mentioned, the randomized clinical trial is a form of experimental research in which the effects of one or more treatments (interventions) are compared with a control "treatment" by randomly assigning study subjects to the groups and measuring differences in effects (outcomes) of the alternative treatments over time. Although its most common use has been to evaluate the effectiveness of medical therapies such as medications and surgical procedures, the RCT can also be used to evaluate other types of interventions.

An RCT has the following characteristics:

- It is a prospective, comparative, longitudinal study involving cohorts of study subjects assigned to alternative treatment groups.
- It is research based on an hypothesized relationship between cause and effect. The hypothesis usually is that the treatment(s) will cause beneficial effects in the treated subjects.
- Study subjects are assigned randomly (by chance alone) to the different treatment groups to control selection bias and to enhance the equivalence (balancing) of the groups in terms of uncontrolled variables that could confound the results (outcomes) by influencing reactions to the treatment.
- As an additional control over biased results in clinical trials of pharmaceuticals, subjects assigned to the control group are given a *placebo*, a pharmacologically inert agent or a standard agent, made to resemble the medication being evaluated in size, shape, and color. Moreover, neither researchers nor subjects know to which group—treatment or control—the subjects are assigned. Known as the *double-blind* or *double-masked* procedure, this technique is a further attempt to make the groups equivalent in everything except the active ingredient in the therapy given to the treatment group. The concept of the pill-placebo "treatment" has relevance to interventions other than medications as a technique for making study conditions comparable for both groups.
- Effects (outcomes) are measured in terms of the statistical significance of the extent to which differences in outcomes between treatment and control groups exceed differences that could occur

by chance alone, i.e., differences that would occur "naturally" in the absence of any real effects from the interventions.

- RCTs are conducted in clinical settings. They reflect the effects of treatments as they are applied and, thus, are clinically relevant.
- RCTs are practical evaluation studies and are intended to answer questions about the effectiveness of therapies and procedures.
- RCTs can be used not only to evaluate new therapies, but also to evaluate the efficacy of existing ones.

How Have They Evolved?

Antecedents of the RCT can even be found in the Bible. The Book of Daniel describes a planned experiment in which the impact of food and water on a person's health was studied (Meinert & Tonascia, 1986). James Lind, a Scottish physician, is credited with one of the earliest experiments using a comparison group. In 1747, aboard ship, he divided 12 patients with scurvy into groups, each given a different "treatment," including lime, lemon, and orange juice which turned out to be efficacious (Lind, 1753). Consequently, the eating of citrus fruits to prevent scurvy became standard practice not only aboard ships, but also as a general health practice.

The importance of using a control group to identify the *placebo effect* was recognized as early as 1799 by the British physician, J. Haygarth. He evaluated the efficacy of metallic rods known as Perkins' Tractors used to stroke the body of people with such conditions as crippling rheumatism, pleurisy, and gout. He also used "fictitious tractors" on a few patients made of wood as a placebo to keep the comparison groups as equal as possible by subjecting all patients to an experimental intervention (Haygarth, 1800). Differences in effects could then be called the treatment effects, and if efficacious, could be credited to the benefits of the metal tractors.

In the early 19th century the basic elements of objective, controlled, and quantitative experiments in the treatment of patients were set forth by P. C.A. Louis (Louis, 1834). These included precise and accurate observations of the phenomena under study, reliable recordings of treatments, and quantitative comparisons of effects on patients. Louis emphasized the importance of *controlled* experiments in which extraneous factors are rigorously suppressed or at least identified, isolated, and accounted for when research findings are interpreted. G. T.

Fechner in the mid-1800s discussed quantitative analyses of experimental research (Fechnet, 1966).

The British statistician R.A. Fisher advocated the use of *randomization* to allocate subjects to different groups in agricultural experiments (Fisher, 1925, 1926; Fisher & MacKenzie, 1923). As conceived by Fisher, assignment of subjects to the comparison groups by chance insures that a treatment "will not be favored or handicapped in successive replications by some extraneous source of variation, known or unknown" (Cochran & Cox, 1950, p. 6).

A major advantage of randomization is that it allows the use of statistical techniques to determine the statistical significance of outcomes; that is, the extent to which outcomes exceed that expected from chance alone (Hill, 1955). In other words, randomization makes it possible to get a valid answer to the question: Are the observed differences in outcomes between the treatment and control groups attributable to treatment or to chance?

Over the years the RCT method has been increasingly applied in the field of health beginning with an evaluation of medication for the treatment of tuberculosis (Amberson, McMahon, & Pinner, 1931). A number of well-publicized RCTs have been conducted in recent years. These have included tests of the Salk vaccine for poliomyelitis, streptomycin for the treatment of tuberculosis, a variety of drugs for cancer therapy, and aspirin for the prevention of myocardial infarction. Many RCTs have been conducted simultaneously in different clinical settings as part of a multicenter approach such as the Multiple Risk Factor Intervention Trial (MR FIT) funded by the National Heart, Lung, and Blood Institute. Therapies for HIV and AIDS have also been investigated in multicenter trials. In Fall 1993 the largest clinical trial ever undertaken was begun, called the Women's Health Initiative (Baker, 1993). Sponsored by the federal government's National Institutes of Health, the 15-year trial will probe causes of diseases and death in midlife and older women.

Although RCTs are applicable to the testing of other interventions besides drugs, the methodological requirements such as control groups, random allocation, placebo, masking, adherence to clinical protocols, and control of attrition, can be adhered to more easily in drug testing than in other types of interventions. Applications of RCTs in nursing have been few and far between, but several examples will be discussed in this chapter.

The RCT Process

An RCT consists of the following activities:

- A plan for the trial is written that specifies the treatment to be tested in detail, including a quantitative statement of effects to be attained by its use and a description of the target population to whom the treatment will be applied.
- Clinically relevant quantitative measures of treatment effects are devised.
- The comparison groups are composed.
- The null hypothesis, which holds that treatment effects will not differ significantly among the groups, is stated. Alternative hypotheses are formulated that state the magnitude of differences in effects that are considered indicative of treatment efficacy.
- A sample of study subjects is recruited from the target population and randomly assigned to comparison groups. A statement of protection of the rights of study subjects is prepared.
- The treatment is applied to one group, or various levels or versions to several groups. The treatment is withheld from one group, the control group, which receives a placebo or standard regimen. Ideally, treatments and placebos should be disguised for both study subjects and researchers.
- After an appropriate amount of time has lapsed, measurements of the effects are taken for the comparison groups, these are subjected to statistical analyses that test for the extent to which differences in effects depart from what is expected to occur by chance alone.

In developing a proposal to use the RCT methodology in nursing, the following questions need to be answered for each major step in the process.

1. *Determine the organization and structure of the project.* What is the project staffing? What is the role of nurses in the project: principal investigator, research coordinator, data collector, advocate for study subjects, implementor of the intervention? How are research tasks assigned, and how do they flow as the project unfolds? How are resources allocated to the major components of the project? Is there an advisory committee to monitor overall performance? Will the project be part of a multicenter research effort?

2. *Define the research problem.* What is the purpose of the research? What will be evaluated? What are the hypotheses: null, alter-

native? Does the research problem rest on any theory? Is there a model for the research?

3. *Define the study population*. What is the population (universe, sampling frame) from whom the sample will be selected and to whom the study findings can be generalized?

4. *Determine eligibility criteria for participation in the study*. What are the eligibility criteria? How do they relate to the definition of the study population?

5. *Decide how to select the sample from the population*. What method will be used to draw the sample from the study population: simple random sample, stratified sample, systematic sample?

6. *Select the method by which sample subjects enter the study*. Will the sample members be entered into the study as a group, or will they be entered sequentially? How will the compliance of study subjects be ensured? How will the rights of subjects be protected? How will risks to the subjects be minimized?

7. *Determine how the comparison groups will be composed*. How is the treatment group defined? What is the nature of the treatment (intervention)? Will there be more than one treatment group, representing different versions (types, levels, intensities) of the treatment? How is the control group defined? What is the nature of the placebo, if any?

8. *Describe how outcomes will be measured*. What measure(s) will be used to evaluate the treatment effects? Over what period of time will measurements be taken? Will the measurements be repeated at predetermined intervals? How will the validity and reliability of the measures be assessed?

9. *Determine what other variables will be measured*. What demographic, socioeconomic, physiologic, psychologic, and other variables will be measured, at baseline and during the study? How will these be related to treatment and outcome variables?

10. *Describe how the safety of the study subjects will be monitored?* What are the risks of participation to the subjects? Are appropriate consent forms used? Are there any side effects of the interventions likely to occur? What are the procedures for altering or modifying the interventions if adverse effects occur?

11. *Determine how the data will be processed*. What computer software will process the data? How will the data be recorded in an appropriate format for computerization? How will the data entry screens be designed? What data entry system will be used: key entry, electronic?

12. *Select the method for analyzing the outcomes.* How will the differences in outcomes be analyzed? What confidence level will be used in testing the statistical significance of the differences? What is the *power* of the test in detecting a significant difference? What does the power of the test indicate about desirable sample size?

13. *Select the sample subjects.* What randomization technique will be used for sample selection? How large a sample is needed to achieve the desired power level? How will drop outs be replaced? How will missing data be addressed?

14. *Allocate the sample subjects to the various comparison group.* What randomization method will be used to assign the subjects to the alternative groups? Will a masking technique (double blind) be used? How can bias effectively be controlled in situations in which the treatment cannot, for all practical purposes, be disguised?

15. *Make baseline measurements.* What are the values for the outcome measures and for other variables of interest at the beginning of the study? Which are important to the analysis of covariance?

16. *Apply and monitor the intervention.* Are the subjects in the treatment group(s) receiving the treatment(s) uniformly and consistently? Are members of the control group receiving a placebo or other alternative treatment? Is the safety of subjects routinely monitored?

17. *Determine the stopping rules.* At what point will the intervention be terminated?

18. *Measure the outcome variables.* What are the values of outcome variables at the end of the study as well as at selected times during the study? What are the values of other relevant variables at these times? How is the quality of the measurements monitored?

19. *Enter the data into the computer.* Are the data properly edited for computer entry? How is the accuracy of data entry monitored?

20. *Analyze the data.* How are the data reduced and summarized? What tests of significance are used? Are they appropriate to the data? What do the tests reveal about the effects of the interventions?

21. *Interpret the findings.* What are the limitations and strengths of the study? Are the differences among comparison groups statistically significant? Are they practically significant? What relevance do the study findings have? Can they be realistically used outside the confines of the study setting? Do the findings contradict or confirm reported findings in other studies? How can the findings be implemented? Are there any recommendations for further research? Does the study have any implications for model and theory development?

22. *Close out the study*. How will the research be terminated in a nondisruptive and orderly fashion? How will the findings be disseminated? How will they be utilized in nursing practice?

To What Kinds of Research Problems Can the RCT be Applied?

The RCT has become closely associated with medical research, primarily in the search for the efficacious treatment of diseases with drugs or surgery or other procedures and technologies. As its name implies, the RCT has a clinical purpose—to determine appropriate therapies for the diagnosis, cure, or alleviation of illnesses.

But this does not mean that applications of experimental designs such as RCTs must be confined to medical or clinical problems. RCTs could also be used to test managerial interventions such as the effects on productivity of different styles of management.

A number of nursing studies have evaluated clinically oriented interventions without the RCT design (Edwards, Herman, Wallace, Pavy, & Harrison-Pavy, 1991). As Wilson (1991, p. 280) remarked, "The dailiness of nursing practice offers an important source of clinically relevant research problems" that could be tested qualitatively as well as quantitatively. Nurse researchers have applied the methodology of qualitative research to an examination of clinical nursing. As already noted, there are major differences between qualitative research methodology and the RCT. Not only is the RCT dependent on quantitative measurement, but its research orientation is the opposite of the qualitative study's which makes observations of the real world and then develops theories—the inductive method. The RCT begins with hypotheses and theories and then tests them in the real world—the deductive approach. RCTs evaluate relationships between dependent and independent variables; the focus of qualitative research is on the behavior of discrete phenomena.

It is possible to conceive of many nursing interventions that could be evaluated through the RCT, or, more precisely, a modified RCT, because it would be very difficult or even impossible to adhere to all of its design requirements. But it is not absolutely essential that a study comply with all requirements to be considered a clinical trial. Adherence to the general features of the RCT, particularly those that address the control of bias, will enhance the validity of all evaluation studies.

The methodology for conducting a clinical trial is highly formalized. There are a number of excellent sources on how to conduct an RCT according to established rules (Friedman, Furberg, & DeMets, 1984; Fleiss, 1986; Meinert & Tonascia, 1986). These books not only provide information on the steps to be followed, but explain how to cope with the problems that arise during the course of the trial. Specialized texts on clinical research in the social and behavioral sciences are also available (Kazdin, 1992).

The proper use of an RCT as a method for doing nursing research raises several important issues. These include: defining the target population; selecting and randomizing the study subjects; managing the RCT; analyzing and interpreting the data; and recognizing the limitations and strengths of the RCT as a methodology for nursing research. These issues are illustrated in the following nursing RCT, the purpose of which was to evaluate early hospital discharge and home follow up of very-low birth weight (VLBW) infants (Brooten et al., 1986).

The study was conducted in the University of Pennsylvania Hospital of infants with very low birthweights (VLBW) of 1,500 grams or less. Thirty-nine VLBW infants were randomly assigned to the treatment group and 40 to the control group. Infants in the control group were kept in hospital until they weighed 2,200 grams, discharged if clinically well and eating satisfactorily. During the hospital stay they received standard care and parents received support and instruction from nursery nurses.

Infants in the treatment group were discharged before they reached 2,200 grams, if clinically well, able to feed by nipple and to maintain body temperature in an open crib, had no serious apnea or bradycardia, and there was an adequate home care environment. On average, this group were discharged 11 days earlier than the control group. The treatment consisted of visits by the nurse during the first week, and at 1, 9, 12, and 18 months. Included in the visits were physical assessment, developmental screening, assessment of parents' coping and care-taking skills, and instruction and counseling regarding infant care. The home health nurse coordinated care with other health care providers.

Data analysis showed no statistically significant differences between the two groups on such outcome measures as rehospitalization rates, episodes of acute care, failure to thrive, or incidences of abuse. The one significant difference was cost of care, which for an early-discharged infant averaged $20,000 less than the control group. The treatment produced the same effects, but with much lower costs. In the face of escalating health care costs and a rising incidence of VLBW infants, this is a indeed a significant finding.

What does this study reveal about using the RCT method to evaluate a nursing program? The first issue is that of generalization of findings.

The Target Population in a RCT

The intention of research using RCTs is to generalize the findings widely. This is quite important as many RCTs evaluate interventions with potential for significant impact on people's health and welfare. The definition of the scope of the population to whom the findings are applicable, called the target population, includes not only the characteristics of its members such as age, sex, and educational attainment, but also its geographic and temporal boundaries. Are the findings to apply only to people who live in warm climates? In the United States? Are they to apply for an indefinite or limited time period?

Problems of generalization are difficult enough in the clinical trials of drugs and other technologies. They are especially challenging in RCTs involving human interventions, such as in nursing, where the "treatment" may be difficult to standardize or even to define. Dissemination of study findings should be unambiguous and uniformly understood and applied. When the results of drug trials are disseminated, the intervention can be expressed in the well-established technical and numbers-laden language of chemical composition and dosages. Dissemination of nursing interventions also requires standardization of terminology and definitions.

Generalizing from a RCT is the same process as generalizing from a descriptive *survey* the purpose of which is to make population estimates from sample data. Good survey procedures require, first, definition of the target population. (Beyond the target population is a larger, hypothetical universe, or, as Hahn and Meeker (1993) define it, a *conceptual population*, for whom the estimates may also be pertinent.)

Next, the *sampling frame* is constructed. The frame is a list, directory, map, or some other source that includes the members of the target population, known as the *sampling units*. To select study subjects a *random* sample is drawn from the sampling frame. (In a random sample each sampling unit has a *known*—greater than zero—probability of being selected in the sample. In a simple, unrestricted sample the probability is equal for all sampling units; in the case of a stratified sample, selection probabilities may not necessarily be equal.) The important thing is that each sampling unit has a definite chance to be included in the sample and that neither researcher nor study subject exerts any influence over selection of sampling units.

Random sampling has two benefits. First, it helps prevent selection of a biased sample, that is, a sample whose responses are not representative of the target population. Second, it allows computation, based on statistical models, of the sampling error (confidence interval) of the sample data.

In the case of the study of the early discharge of VLBW infants, as is true for many RCTs, the findings cannot, strictly speaking, be statistically extrapolated from the sample as can survey data based on random samples. The study was done in one, nonrandomly selected hospital. What, then, is the target population? Is it all hospitals? Medical centers only? All hospitals in Pennsylvania? Or is the target population VLBW infants? (All VLBW infants? In Pennsylvania? In the one hospital?) What then can be done with the findings? Are they really limited to the infants in the study? If that were the case, the cost-effectiveness of RCTs would be extremely low.

However, there is an important difference between a descriptive survey and an RCT when it comes to making generalizations of findings. An RCT investigates *relationships* between treatments and outcomes; the data that will be projected to the target population are the *effects* of these relationships. As Deming has stated (1975), an RCT is an *analytical* study in which the focus is on future hypothetical performance (effects). If the effects are statistically and substantively significant there is a motivation to generalize them widely, even if a target population was not defined from which study subjects were randomly selected. What really is important in making a convincing generalization of the benefits of the intervention tested, as in the case of the VLBW infant study, is to apply the clinical knowledge and expertise of the researcher to the *interpretation* of the findings.

Two recent developments help to strengthen generalization of results from an RCT: *multicenter trials* and *meta-analysis*. A multicenter trial is the replication of an RCT in several different settings to increase the level of confidence in research findings. Multicenter trials enlarge the sample of subjects and provide more definitive findings. The study of aspirin as a preventative for myocardial infarction is an example of a large multicenter RCT (Aspirin Myocardial Infarction Study Research Group, 1980). Multicenter trials, however, are difficult to manage, increase costs, and require considerable coordination. Meta-analysis is a relatively inexpensive way of simulating a multicenter trial by combining secondary data from a number of RCTs and statistically analyzing them as if the studies were true replications.

Selecting and Randomizing the Study Subjects

Perhaps more than any other type of research design, a clinical trial requires much commitment and involvement from its subjects. RCTs are longitudinal studies extending over fairly lengthy time periods. The study of VLBW infants spanned more than 2 years. Also, RCTs can require some kind of intrusive treatment: a potent drug, an experimental surgical procedure, or exposure to a new kind of care program. How much easier it is to be a study subject in a survey in which data collection consists of responding to a brief questionnaire or interview.

Selecting the study subjects for an RCT and randomly allocating them to the various comparison groups includes the following steps:

1. Determine eligibility criteria for inclusion in the study;
2. Determine sample size;
3. Select the sample of study subjects; and
4. Determine method for randomly allocating subjects to the different groups.

1. Determine Eligibility Criteria

Determining eligibility for entering a subject into an RCT requires a clear definition of the target population. For example, in the home health care study the target population was very low-birthweight infants defined as 1,500 grams or less (Brooten et al., 1986). However, not all infants born in this weight class were considered as potential subjects. It was believed too risky to have infants with complications such as apnea or bradycardia undergo an experimental type of care involving early discharge. Also, some infants were eliminated because of problems in the home or parents' refusals to participate.

Thus, the process of determining eligibility for participation generates attrition of subjects who, although meeting the most essential eligibility criteria, do not enter the study. Some potential subjects simply refuse to participate. Obtaining informed consent from every participant is a requirement prior to entry into the study.

Attrition from the study may require redefinition of the target population before the data are generalized. The home health care study may have initially defined the population as all VLBW infants, but it was later modified to include only healthy infants from functional home environments. The fact that study subjects are not *randomly* selected from a defined target population and some subjects are lost through attrition increase difficulties in generalizing the data.

2. Determine Sample Size

There are two ways of determining sample size for RCTs. One is called *fixed* sample size and the other, *sequential sampling*. In the fixed sample size design the investigator specifies the number of sample subjects to be included before data collection begins. In the sequential design, sample size is not specified in advance. Instead, subjects are added to the sample progressively until *effect size* exceeds a preselected value.

Sequential sampling is potentially more cost-effective than fixed sampling because it minimizes the sample size needed to adequately test the study hypotheses (Armitage, 1975). Keeping sample size to a minimum is especially important in longitudinal studies. However, the sequential approach is efficient only when significant effects are expected to occur in a short time, enabling data collection to be ended sooner than if sample size were fixed in advance. It is unlikely that a sequential sampling design would have been helpful in the home health study because of the long delay between treatment and outcomes.

Analysis of power. A statistical technique, called *power analysis*, can be used to determine sample size needed to reduce the chance of *not* finding significant effects when they are really there (the so-called Type II error). However, practical considerations are also important in determining sample size. These include availability of study subjects, time scheduled for the study, resources on hand, and amount of descriptive data desired. In addition to power, sample size determination considers the design of the study: the number and nature of comparison groups, outcome measures to be used and whether scales are qualitative or quantitative, effect size considered to be clinically significant stated hypotheses, statistical techniques to test the hypotheses, and level of significance utilized (Lachin, 1981).

To clarify the concept of power it is necessary to begin with the study hypotheses. Theoretically, every study that tests for the statistical significance of differences in treatment effects between control and treatment groups poses two hypotheses: the *null hypothesis*, which states that a statistically significant difference between the measure of effects *does not* exist, and the *alternative hypothesis*, which states that a significant difference *does* exist. The amount or percentage of acceptable (clinically relevant) difference (the effect size) may be stated in the alternative hypothesis.

A statistical test of significance determines the extent to which the sample effect size accurately reflects the population effect size. The test tells us the *probability* that the sample value is the true population value. In comparing outcome measures in an RCT the sample value that is tested is the *difference* in outcomes between treatment and control groups: the effect size. The null hypothesis (null means zero in German) states that no (zero) difference exists in the population. Thus, if our statistical test of the difference between the two measures is not significant—that is, the size of the difference is not larger than the underlying statistical model for the test tells us can occur by chance alone at the level of significance we have chosen—we accept the null hypothesis and reject the alternative hypothesis. Conversely, if the difference between the measures *exceeds* the value expected at our level of significance, the null hypothesis is rejected and the alternative hypothesis is accepted.

Two types of errors can occur in this process. The size of these errors and the probability of their occurrence depend on the level of significance chosen for the statistical testing, the type of test used including whether the test is one- or two-sided, and the number of subjects on whom the test is based. The errors are also related to the impact of the intervention: the statistical significance of a small effect (small difference between treatment and control group outcomes) is harder to detect than is a large impact, particularly when samples are small.

In the *Type I* error the null hypothesis is falsely *rejected* and the alternative hypothesis accepted. This occurs when it is concluded from the sample that the difference in outcomes between the treatment and control groups (the effect size) *is* statistically significant when a real difference does not truly exist for the population. The Type I error leads to the false conclusion that the intervention was efficacious.

In the *Type II* error the opposite situation occurs: the null hypothesis is falsely *accepted* and the alternative hypothesis rejected. This occurs when it is concluded that the difference in treatment effects is *not* statistically significant when, in fact, a real difference does exist in the population. A Type II error leads to the false conclusion that the intervention was not efficacious.

The statistical significance of an effect size increases as the size of the sample increases. It is obvious that if the entire population were studied, any effect size, no matter how small, would be statistically significant. The statistical significance of large effect sizes is easier to detect with smaller samples than the significance of small effects.

The probability of making a Type I error, called *alpha*, is the level of significance selected for the statistical test. A level of 0.05 means that the chance of falsely rejecting the null hypothesis—concluding that the treatment was efficacious when it really was not—is 5 out of 100. Thus, the probability of *not* making a Type I error is 1 minus alpha, in this case 0.95, which is called the *confidence level*.

The probability of making a Type II error is called *beta*. The value of 1 minus beta, which is the probability of *not* making a Type II error, is called the *power* of the statistical test. A power of 0.80 is considered a desirable level (Kramer & Thiemann, 1987; Cohen, 1990).

Power can be computed with available computer software. Statistical graphs are also available that show the power level for different effect sizes according to the statistical test used and whether it was one or two-tailed, sample size, and alpha level. (Friedman, Furberg, & DeMets, 1984; Stuart & Ord, 1991). Power increases for a given effect size and alpha level when size of sample is increased.

In actual practice some RCTs do not calculate power in determining sample size. (It is not clear from the article on the home health study that power was analyzed.) Practical rather than statistical considerations often dictate sample size. Samples of size 30 are quite common, based more on conventional wisdom than on assessment of power. Proposals are often criticized by grant review bodies because of the absence of power analysis. It cannot be reiterated too strongly, however, that power analysis does not guarantee a good study. High power cannot in any way compensate for poor data.

3. Select the Sample

The home health study reported that nearly 40,000 VLBW infants are born each year in the United States (Brooten et al., 1986). In a sense, this is the target population for the study. During the period of the study at the Hospital of the University of Pennsylvania, 136 infants were born in this weight class, although not all were eligible. Fifty-seven were excluded for various reasons: 6 died, 34 were in poor health, and 17 were from problem families who refused to participate, which left 79 eligible. Mothers and other caretakers were also considered as sample members, and, in a sense, they were, although measurement of treatment effects was focused on the infants. Obviously, these were not randomly selected samples.

4.   Determine Method of Random Allocation

Comparison groups: A key feature of RCTs is comparison of the effects of different treatments including effects of nontreatment. The eligible sample is divided into two groups: the *treatment* group receiving the intervention and the *control* group from whom the intervention is withheld. An RCT may also have multiple treatment groups defined according to different levels, dosages, or versions of the intervention, such as a drug by mouth or intravenously.

In the home care RCT, infants in the treatment group were discharged early to home care—the intervention under study—while the control group received conventional nursery care. As in many nondrug RCTs, the double-blind technique would not have worked. The researchers obviously knew the group assignment of each subject.

Controlling bias: An RCT in which the double blind is not used because it is not possible to mask the intervention is called "unblinded" or "unmasked." Trials in which the investigators but not the study subjects know which group a subject is placed is called "single-blinded." It can be argued that a single-blinded trial is as good as a double-blinded one, since it would be possible to measure the impact of the "Hawthorne effect" by determining how much of the effect size is due to subjects' reactions to the act of participating in the study. However, it has been shown that, without double blinding, investigators may compensate for the withholding of the intervention from control group subjects by providing extra care that normally would not be provided, thus distorting outcomes even if the Hawthorne effect is controlled (Friedman, Furberg, & DeMets, 1986).

Arguably, it is desirable to use the double blind technique in all RCTs, but it is impossible to do so unless a masked placebo can effectively be employed. Without one, the investigator must depend on analysis of the data to sort out biases.

Historical control group: Not all RCTs employ control groups to which study subjects are assigned randomly. An alternate design is to use data from secondary sources as the control such as from previous studies and from databases, for example, such as Duke University's *Cardiovascular Disease Databank* (U. S. General Accounting Office,

1992). Another source of data is patient records maintained by health agencies.

Studies that use secondary data in place of an actual control group are called "historical control" studies. Dispensing with the control group means that all subjects are assigned to the treatment group. Their outcomes are then compared to the outcomes from the secondary sources, which could include studies previously carried out in the same research center as well as earlier exploratory and pilot studies. It is fortuitous if results of a meta-analysis are available to serve as a "control group."

Studies that use randomly assigned control groups are known as studies with *internal* controls (Bailar, Louis, Lavor, & Polanski, 1984). Studies without control groups are simply labeled studies without controls. Studies that use historical data as controls are called studies with *external* controls, but they lack randomization.

Historical data that could be used as external controls can be assembled in the literature review phase of the study. Using these data in place of a control group has several advantages. By eliminating the control group the researcher can reduce the costs of the study and simplify the management. The savings could be used to enlarge the size of the treatment group. Also, in trials of therapies expected to be clinically effective, the researcher may not feel that it is in the subject's best interest to withhold an efficacious treatment until the study is completed (Gehan & Freireich, 1974). This was the situation in the release of the drug AZT to persons with AIDS before it was completely evaluated.

The use of secondary data as a substitute for a control group has several limitations. One is data quality. This is less of an issue if the data have been subjected to a meta-analysis. Another problem is comparability. Are the study subjects really similar? The interventions? The outcome measures? Also, there is the question of the appropriateness of statistical analysis of mixed data from independent studies. Similar problems are faced in conducting a meta-analysis.

Concurrent studies: It may be possible to dispense with a control group if comparable data are available from ongoing studies. Multicenter studies have the potential to provide data on outcomes from a number of separate studies that could be considered controls.

Crossover designs: Although recently applied to the RCT method, crossover designs have been used in social science research for many years. In a crossover design, study subjects are members of a control *and* a treatment group, essentially serving as their own controls. The subject first receives a treatment or a control, depending on randomized assignment, and later receives the alternative intervention. Because in drug trials the design removes biologic variation, a smaller sample can be used without reducing the power of the statistical tests. However, the design has its drawbacks, one of which is the possible carryover of the effects of treatment from one phase to the other (Louis, Lavori, Bailar, & Polansky, 1984). An extreme form of the crossover design is a randomized trial in which the sample consists of a single subject (Guyatt, Sackett, Taylor, Chong, Roberts, & Pugsley, 1986).

Random allocation techniques: There are two main types of allocation techniques. One type, called "fixed allocation," allocates the assignment of sample subjects to either treatment or control groups with a probability that is specified prior to assignment, and the probability remains unchanged during the study. The other type is called "adaptive allocation" in which the probability changes during the course of the study in order to deliberately balance the groups in terms of baseline characteristics of subjects or their responses to treatment. The latter approach, which is most applicable in the testing of therapeutic interventions, may assign a subject to the same group as the last subject if the response to the treatment was successful. The intent is to maximize the number of subjects receiving an efficacious treatment (Zelen, 1969).

In fixed allocation the mechanics of randomly allocating the subjects to different groups are similar to the techniques used in survey sampling. In *simple unrestricted randomization* a coin toss can be used to determine the allocation as each sample subject enters the study: heads to treatment, tails to control. If there are more than two groups, random numbers are used to make the random assignments. A disadvantage of this type of assignment is that the study will end up with different numbers of subjects in each comparison group. To circumvent this problem the technique of *blocked randomization* is used to allocate the subjects by controlling the numbers in each group. *Stratified randomization* goes one step further by not only controlling the the number of subjects in each group, but also balancing their characteristics by assignment according to what the investigator believes to be important baseline characteristics, such as age, sex, ethnicity, and so on.

5. Other Types of Experimental Designs

Variations of the basic experimental design have been developed to increase efficiency and improve data quality (Cochran & Cox, 1950;

Fisher, 1947; Mason, Gunst, & Hess, 1989). These designs originated in agricultural and biological experiments, and some do not transfer easily to experimentation with humans. The *latin square* design and its variations—*Graeco-latin squares, lattices*—are essentially methods of stratified, or more precisely, *blocked* randomization that are useful in reducing random error when the treatment consists of more than one version or level, such as testing several different drugs in one clinical trial for the reduction of hypertension.

The *factorial* design is useful in testing the effects of a number of different factors (variables) simultaneously. The treatments consist of all *combinations* that can be formed from the different factors. One factor could be two different types of drugs for the treatment of hypertension, and the other, two different dosage levels. This is called a 2 by 2 factorial experiment, yielding 4 treatment combinations that would be tested simultaneously in the clinical trial. This can be done within a crossover design, so that much information can be elicited from just a few subjects. The factorial is an interesting design that as yet has had few uses in nursing research, although there have been a number of nonexperimental studies in which multiple independent variables, not necessarily in combination, were examined.

Managing an RCT

Conducting an RCT is a major undertaking. Unlike other forms of research there is no such thing as a *small* RCT. A fairly large sample of study subjects is needed to attain a respectable level of power. Data are collected longitudinally, requiring repeated measurements to be made with high accuracy over a long time period. And, most importantly, an RCT has to be managed very tightly and must strictly adhere to the research design as originally conceived. Consequently, RCTs require a tightly controlled organizational structure and well developed operating procedures (Melink & Whitacre, 1991).

A clinical trial requires considerable paperwork. The organization and management of an RCT are described in various documents. A *study proposal* is the document submitted to obtain funding. It contains the study objectives, its significance, review of previous studies, technical approach, and resources required including facilities, personnel, and money. The proposal attempts to put the study in its best light because it must compete with other proposals. The *manual of operations* is an internal document prepared after the study is approved and funded. It is primarily used for the day-to-day management of the study, containing a detailed description of the study's organizational structure, assignment of tasks, and its purposes, policies, and procedures. The *study protocol* is a less detailed statement of the aims, background, design, and methodology that serves primarily as an explanatory prospectus for study participants and members of the scientific community.

Once the RCT begins there must be strict adherence to the design and methodology as spelled out in the manual of operations and protocol. That no one is allowed to "wing it" assures comparability of results, especially important in multicenter trials.

Three aspects of managing an RCT will be discussed: staffing, quality control of the data, and troubleshooting.

Staffing

An RCT cannot conceivably be a one-person operation. Publications of results of RCTs usually have multiple authors, indicating that a large staff was involved. The home health study; for example, had 8 authors. Staffing of an RCT usually includes a principal investigator as its head to provide overall leadership for the project; a study director responsible for the day-to-day management, a study coordinator to provide liaison between study and clinical setting and with other centers in multicenter trials; study investigators; data collectors; data processors; and data analysts.

Consultants such as statisticians are needed because of the many statistical tasks that must be accomplished, i.e., constructing the randomization procedure, analyzing power and determining sample size, designing measuring instruments, and performing statistical tests. Other consultants, including pharmacologists, physiologists, psychometricians, and computer programmers, also provide technical expertise. In short, an RCT requires a complex blending of knowledge and skills.

Nurses have had many different roles in clinical trials. Nurses have been principal investigators in the rare RCT that tested a nursing intervention. Nurses have also been project directors, senior investigators, and data collectors in non-nursing RCTs. An increasingly important role for nurses is the recruiting, screening, making baseline assessments of subjects, and overseeing the protection of subject safety and rights. Also, the role of study coordinator is frequently taken by nurses.

An RCT is a team effort, requiring a mix of skills and coordination of many tasks and responsibilities. Because of extensive staffing, costs of conducting an RCT are high, but are justified when therapies with the potential for improving the health of large numbers of people are evaluated. This leaves little room for support of RCTs to investigate "smaller" problems, and less costly research approaches must be sought. (Adams, McCall, Gray, Orza, & Chalmers, 1992).

Quality Control of Data

Data are collected at many different stages of an RCT. Before interventions are introduced, baseline measurements are taken of the sample subjects as they are enrolled. Measures of the effects of the interventions—the outcome variables—are taken in repeated measurements during the study and at the end of the data collection phase. The home health study required continuous data collection on episodes of hospitalization, acute care visits, health status of infants, and costs.

Quality control of data includes a number of tasks. First, all measures must be clearly defined and assessed for validity; relevant data collection instruments must be selected from existing sources or created by the researchers; all instruments must be pretested and reliability of instruments assessed; and procedures must be established for maintaining accurate and consistent data collection. Then, after data are collected, they must be edited for completeness and accuracy and made ready for data entry and computer processing. Missing data is an especially troublesome problem requiring special attention. Too much missing data threatens the validity of results.

Control of data quality can be ensured by several simple techniques. First, all data collectors, and, in fact, all key study personnel, should receive thorough training in the proper use of data collection instruments. Second, reliability checks should be made on the data on a sample basis, using independent auditors. Third, data can be checked for consistency and accuracy by running some statistical tests on a spot check basis as they are collected. Waiting until the data collection stage is completed to begin the data analysis is perilous. Data should be checked against similar data from previous studies. The expertise of consultants can be enlisted to review interim data for clinical relevance. The method of sequential sampling lends itself quite nicely to this type of quality control check. Finally, a quality control committee should be established within the project with ongoing responsibility for monitoring data quality.

Maintenance of data quality is important for all types of research. Data quality is especially important in RCTs because the validity and usefulness of findings are completely dependent on quantitative measures. Also, important decisions may be based on RCT results that can affect the delivery and costs of health care to large numbers of people.

Troubleshooting

In studies as complex and time-consuming as RCTs problems will undoubtedly arise (Corman & Davidson, 1992). Three fairly common difficulties are: unbalanced comparison groups, sample attrition, and modification of the intervention.

Unbalanced Groups

A goal of randomization is to obtain comparison groups that are equivalent in terms of important characteristics, but this is by no means assured. Treatment group subjects can turn out to have different characteristics than control group subjects, affecting their reaction to the treatment. In the home health care study it is possible that an uncontrolled variable helped the early discharged infants respond well to the care they received. If this variable is identified early on, it can be controlled by using a blocked design that randomizes according to predetermined strata.

However, even stratified randomization may not balance the groups because a hidden factor could affect outcomes. And the further the assignment process moves away from unrestricted randomization, the greater the danger of selection bias; i.e., study subjects having a greater potential for favorable response to the intervention are assigned to the treatment rather than the control group by the investigators, unconsciously or perhaps even deliberately (Wahrendorf & Blettner, 1985). This may not necessarily be done to "cook" the data, but to make available what is believed to be an efficacious intervention as soon as possible.

One technique for making groups comparable is *covariate adjustment*. This technique balances the groups statistically using baseline data to minimize the effects of differences in important characteristics. But even attempts to balance groups may miss an important confounding variable. It is necessary to keep an open mind during all stages of the study, especially when the data are being interpreted, and being aware of the possibility that study outcomes may be at least partially caused by factors other than the intervention. Moreover, it is important to remember that an RCT, regardless of how large its sample may be, is essentially a sample of one trial. The sample is enlarged when the findings are confirmed (or denied) by other studies. It is unwise to make major decisions on the basis of a single study.

Sample Attrition

As in any longitudinal study in which the study subjects are humans, the problem of retention until data collection is completed is challenging (Given, Given, & Coyle, 1985). Some subjects die, a not unusual occurrence if the sample is composed of older people. Other subjects may quit for a variety of reasons. Still others may not consistently comply with the protocol, e.g., not take the treatment as scheduled. Another possibility is that a subject will try to crossover from the treatment to the control group because of displeasure with the treatment, or, conversely, from the control to the treatment group to obtain the assumed benefits of the intervention.

Action should be taken to control attrition, since it can seriously unbalance the comparison groups. One of the first safeguards is to oversample to provide a cushion for later losses. Balance of comparison groups will be maintained if the characteristics of the dropouts do not follow a systematic pattern, for example, the dropouts are not predominantly older than the stayers. The sample can also be adjusted retrospectively, if the sample was large enough to begin with, by eliminating from the analysis any subject whose characteristics matched a dropout from the other group, a drastic solution to the attrition problem.

The best solution to the attrition problem is to design the study to be as "subject-friendly" as possible and to make every effort to obtain a high degree of subject compliance. Minimizing the time of involvement in the study helps in reducing attrition, as does the simplicity and ease with which the intervention is applied. Techniques for maximizing compliance include avoidance of selection of subjects who have problems that could interfere with their participation, such as living long distances from the study site; keeping the subjects informed about all aspects of the study (except which group they are in if the study is blinded); involving the subject's spouse or another family member in the study; making all contacts with study staff as pleasant as possible; and providing monetary compensation or other reward for participation.

Modification of the Treatment

In clinical trials of drugs it is easier to standardize the treatment and maintain its consistency throughout the study than in other kinds of interventions. In the home health study, how were the nursing visits to the early discharged infants standardized, and how were they kept consistent from one time to another and among different infants? Theoretically, to keep the intervention consistent, the same nurse should have made all the visits. It appears from the study report that three nurses, one full-time and two part-time provided the follow up care in the homes. It can be assumed that the care was reasonably comparable.

Modification of treatment is more likely to be due to subjects than to researchers. In drug trials, subjects may deviate from the protocol because of illness, dissatisfaction with the treatment, or other reasons. In the home health study, opportunities for deviation from the treatment by both infants and their caretakers were numerous during the 18-month period of observation. Solutions to this problem include the aforementioned procedures for gaining patient compliance and monitoring by investigators of the consistency of treatment. If treatment deviations are pronounced, the data for the subjects should either be eliminated from the analysis or analyzed separately (Rabeneck, Viscoli, & Horwitz, 1992). As in the case of dropouts the latter procedure is to be preferred, especially when the samples are small. Loss of power would be considerable if the sample were to be even further reduced in size.

Analyzing and Interpreting Data from an RCT

The analysis of data from an RCT is fairly cut-and-dried. The statistical hypotheses, level of statistical significance for testing the differences between treatment and control groups, and method(s) for testing the differences are all decided in advance of data collection. After the data are collected they are processed and analyzed to answer the question: Is there a statistically significant difference in outcomes between the treatment and control groups? If there is a significant difference, then the conclusion is that the treatment probably *caused* the difference, because all other variables were equalized for the two groups and only the treatment was varied.

At least as important as the statistical significance of outcomes is their clinical significance (Le Fort, 1993). A difference can be statistically significant, but have no clinical importance. The determination of clinical importance, which can also be called practical or substantive importance, occurs after the statistical analysis. This process is known as *interpreting* the data. Its validity depends on the expertise, knowledge, and skills of the interpreter.

Interpretation occurs when it is determined whether or not the study findings are worth generalizing. If so, the characteristics of the target population to whom the sample findings are projected are described and the temporal and spatial boundaries of the generalization are specified.

The conclusions drawn from statistical analysis are based on mathematical laws of probability. The correctness of these conclusions are a matter of *internal validity*, whereas interpretation that extends beyond statistical inference is a different kind of inference, "one that draws on our knowledge of the phenomena under investigation, whether they are smoking habits, income, health status, or whatever. Now we must be concerned with the *external validity* of the conclusions" (Moses, 1985, p. 896).

The home health study found no significant differences between treatment and control groups on any of the outcome measures except cost. Cost was substantially lower for early-discharged infants, a conclusion that has a great deal of practical significance, especially since early discharge had no adverse effects on health.

But many studies end with no statistically significant findings, much to the disappointment of the researchers who expected that their treatment would produce good results. However, nonsignificant findings can be as important and as clinically relevant as significant ones. They can prevent treatment changes that are not good or maybe even harmful.

If the intervention is believed to be beneficial and there is strong motivation for the data to definitively reveal the impact, a number of techniques can be used to increase the likelihood of obtaining statistically significant and, in turn, clinically relevant results in an RCT as well as in all types of evaluative and causal research (U. S. General Accounting Office, 1992):

- Increase the *power* of the test by using larger samples, more balanced samples, designs that reduce variability, and more sensitive statistical tests, including the use of one-sided tests whenever they can be appropriately applied.

- Employ response measures that are highly sensitive to the interventions being tested. These measures should be operationally defined and clinically meaningful. In general, quantitative scales, like physiologic measures, have greater sensitivity than qualitative scales.
- Use interventions likely to have a strong effect on outcome measures. In drug trials dosages can be increased to the limits of safety in order to increase the potential for a significant response. However, to the extent possible, interventions should simulate real world treatments as closely as possible. Unrealistic interventions have limited generalizeability. Moreover, interventions should be standardized and capable of being precisely replicated.

The importance of statistical significance is clear. Without it, causality, if only for the sample subjects, cannot be claimed. Without proof of causality, a clinical trial would be merely a costly, sterile exercise. It seems unlikely that an RCT would be undertaken if the researchers did not believe the intervention would be effective.

But findings that the intervention was ineffective are valuable, too. This stimulates continuation of the search for therapies that are truly beneficial. Also, it is important that an RCT reveal all negative side effects of an intervention. In the home health study, one possible side effect might have been psychological trauma to early-discharged infants. These effects may possibly have remained undetected until after the study was closed. Or, this side effect could have been reversed: infants remaining in the hospital longer could be more traumatized because of negative effects of the hospital environment.

In any case, RCTs should be conducted with the utmost objectivity. Even though a researcher favors the intervention and hopes for its success, the null hypothesis must be given a fair and unbiased test.

Strengths and Limitations of the RCT Methodology

As has been indicated throughout this discussion, there are negative and positive sides to the RCT methodology that can be summarized as follows:

Strengths

- Considered the gold standard of studies that aim to test the effectiveness of therapies, an RCT, using an experimental design, provides an objective approach to the evaluation of causal relationships.
- The RCT provides a mechanism for systematically controlling extraneous variables that can bias study findings.
- Randomization and quantitative outcome measures permit use of a large assortment of powerful statistical techniques to test the significance of data. Results of tests can be disseminated in an objective and widely understood language.
- RCTs can be applied to a variety of interventions, not only to drugs and other medical therapies.
- RCTs are based on well-defined protocols that fully describe all major characteristics of the study including clear definitions of dependent and independent variables. RCTs are usually so well standardized they can easily be replicated in different settings.

Limitations

- RCTs cannot be used for many problems that have to be studied in a different way, using animal subjects or secondary data; for example, studies that involve trauma to the treatment group.
- RCTs are expensive, requiring a large staff and much data processing.
- The RCT process is quite intricate and demanding. It could be called "fussy." The mechanics of randomization and blinding require strict attention to procedural details. There is no room for flexibility, creativity, and expansiveness as in qualitative research.
- A clinical trial cannot be completed in a short time. Several years may be required before follow up of subjects can be concluded and the study terminated.
- The focus of an RCT is typically quite narrow and the results provide only a limited advancement of basic knowledge. The primary purpose is to evaluate an intervention and not to contribute to theory or model development.
- Sample size in RCTs is frequently small. Many studies that employ very small samples do not assess the power of the statistical tests used and, consequently, are open to Type II errors.

- Strictly speaking, statistical generalizations of data from an RCT should not extend beyond the sample studied. Clinical judgement and expertise must be brought to bear on the interpretation of the results in order to extrapolate to a population or universe beyond the sample.
- An RCT can be quite intrusive on study subjects. Ethical issues must be considered, and informed consent and statements of the rights of subjects are essential.
- RCTs are seen by many nurse researchers as applicable only to the evaluation of medical therapies. Some believe that all clinical trials are based on the medical model. Some even call them sexist because only rarely have women served as principal investigators of an RCT.

Some Examples of Non-medical RCTs

Increasingly, the RCT methodology is being applied to the evaluation of nonmedical interventions and programs (Norman, Gadaleta, & Griffin, 1991; Sampselle & Delancey, 1992). Despite the many difficulties that accompany these applications in which the intervention consists wholly or in part of human behavior, as in the home health study, researchers are recognizing that only through the RCT approach can the impact of extraneous variables be effectively controlled.

An interesting example of a modified RCT is a study conducted in Denmark in which 285 randomly selected subjects 75 years of age and over were visited every 3 months (the intervention) and their health status was assessed and advice provided on sources of health and social services if they were deemed necessary (Hendriksen, Lund, & Stromgard, 1984). Twelve visits were made. In the final 3 months of the study a randomly selected control group of 287 people of the same age and sex were visited to determine episodes of hospitalization (outcome measure) that were compared (admission rates) to the treatment group. The data showed that there were fewer admissions to hospitals in the treatment group. One methodological question about this study is whether it is a true RCT, as the treatment and control groups apparently were composed at different time periods by a process of random sampling and not, strictly speaking, by random allocation. Other questions include lack of blinding and absence of a placebo.

In another example a study was made of prenatal and postpartum home visits by nurses in which a broad range of educational and support services were provided (Olds, Henderson, Tatelbaum, & Chamberlin, 1986). Pregnant women who had no previous live births and had one or more risk factors such as young age, single-parent status, or low income, were recruited and randomly assigned to one of four study groups. One group, designated the control group and consisting of 90 subjects, received no prenatal services. The main treatment group, consisting of 116 subjects, received prenatal and postnatal home visits by nurses as well as free transportation to local clinics for prenatal and well-child care. The other two treatment groups, each with about 100 subjects, either received no postnatal visits or were provided free transportation to the clinic and no visits at all. Outcomes as measured by birthweight and length of gestation were most favorable for the group receiving both pre- and postnatal home visits. Again, the absence of blinding in the RCT, which can bias the outcomes, presents a problem when researchers attempt to generalize findings. Moreover, as described by Corman and Davidson (1992), a limitation of many RCTs is the hidden assumption of common etiology and pathogenesis among study subjects. That is, the explicit assumption in this RCT is that low birth weight and prematurity are due to the same cause in every subject, namely, inadequate prenatal care, when, in fact, for some patients there may be other significant reasons for these problems.

Still another RCT in the area of home health care was reported on service for acute stroke patients (Wade, Langton-Hewer, Skilbeck, Bainton, & Burns-Cox, 1985). For the treatment group, consisting of 440 acute stroke patients, staff provided supplementary care in the patients' homes; the 417 patients in the control group received regular care which did not include services in the home. No differences were found in three outcome measures: hospitalization rates, social and emotional adjustment to the stroke, and functional capability of the patients. The researchers, obviously disappointed with their results, attributed lack of impact of the intervention to lack of random allocation of study subjects to treatment and control groups as well as absence of blinding, although blind assessments were considered but were unworkable. Because of the lack of random assignment, the authors speculate that perhaps control group patients came from more supportive homes, as well as on the existence of other imbalances in the composition of the study groups that could have biased the outcomes.

A number of RCTs of nurse interventions in areas other than home care have been reported; a large proportion of these have appeared in British journals. Perhaps the government-run health care system in the United Kingdom stimulates experimentation in nursing roles (Levine, Leatt, & Poulton, 1993). For example, an RCT was reported of nurse therapy for neuroses (Ginsberg, Marks, & Waters, 1984). In one group, 22 neurotic patients were assigned to behavioral psychotherapy from a nurse therapist; in another group, 28 patients received therapy from general practitioners. At the end of a year the study found that the clinical outcome of the nurse-treated patients was significantly better than for those treated by general practitioners. Also, costs were lower for the nurse treated group. However, as the authors of the report caution, the findings cannot be extrapolated too widely without further study because of the small sample and other limitations of the study design, including, as has been said about RCTs in which the intervention is a human service, absence of a placebo, lack of blinding, and variability in the intervention (Crawford, 1992).

Other interventions evaluated in RCTs have included catheter tunneling and a nutrition nurse (Keohane et al., 1983), home uterine monitoring (Grimes & Schultz, 1992), pressure sore treatment (David, 1982), transparent polyurethane IV dressings (Popovsky & Ilstrup, 1986), and the Leboyer approach to childbirth (Nelson, Enkin, Saigal, Bennett, Milner, & Sackett, 1980). As these studies make abundantly clear, interventions that can be evaluated through the RCT method are varied and can have a meaningful nursing content.

The Role of Nurses in Clinical Trials

Nurses are fulfilling significant roles in RCTs that do not necessarily have a nursing content (Guy, 1991; Hubbard, 1982; Willems, 1990). These roles include the following:

Patient educator. Patient education is a collaborative effort between the principal investigator and other members of the research team, including the clinical nurse. The treatment regimen provides the source of information for communicating details of the intervention to the patient. In drug trials, if information is available about possible side effects, the nurse communicates this to the patient with the caution that not all side effects may have yet been identified. Study goals and the process of random assignment are discussed with the patient.

Caregiver. Nursing care of the patient involves assessment, planning, intervention, and evaluation. In an RCT the roles of several different nurses interact: primary nurse, clinical research nurse, and clinical nurse specialist. The primary nurse participates in the plan for the patient's nursing care. The clinical nurse specialist can help to develop a plan for addressing possible side effects. The clinical research nurse's observations about the patients after treatment can help to document any toxicities (Dracup, 1987). A problem that can arise is overloading the primary nurse with research responsibilities (Johansen, Mayer, & Hoover, 1991). Proper attention must be given to the patient care workload in an RCT and the adequacy of staffing to meet that workload.

Patient advocate. The primary nurse caregiver in clinical trials is the patients' advocate and is responsible for seeing that their rights are upheld. The clinical research nurse helps patients define their goals and purposes for participating. The research nurse assists patients who withdraw do so with minimal friction. The research nurse also plays a key role in securing and maintaining patient compliance during the study. This is a most important role (Stichele, 1991). Noncompliance is perhaps the single largest category of problems in conducting an RCT and can lead to its failure.

Coordinator. The research nurse coordinates care and the study protocol. This nurse is responsible for coordinating a patient's care with other involved units such as the pharmacy and laboratory.

Administrator. Nurses' administrative functions include: defining functions and responsibilities, communicating, making decisions, and identifying goals to monitor progress (Abdellah, 1991).

Researcher. In this role, which varies from one study to another, the nurse may be involved in designing the protocol, collecting data, and interpreting, disseminating, and utilizing the findings.

The Future of the RCT Methodology in Nursing Research

Because nurses will continue to play an important role in future clinical trials outside the arena of nursing, the question is: What is the future of the RCT in research that is fully grounded in nursing? A careful weighing of the strengths and weaknesses of the randomized clinical trial methodology suggests that there is a place for it, though perhaps limited, in future nursing research. In some important respects nursing research is becoming more clinically oriented. At the same time increased attention is being focused on the nursing role in health promotion and disease prevention. Also, as the home health study clearly showed, nursing can play an important role in promoting cost-effective health care. In all of these areas there are conceivably a large number of nursing interventions that could be tested, if not in a full-fledged RCT, then in a less costly and simpler design that could be called a modified or quasi-RCT. This is similar to a quasi-experiment that eases some of the methodological requirements of an experiment, yet produces useful data (Cook & Campbell, 1979). There are limits, however, as to how far a quasi-RCT should stray from the ideal model before the validity of results deteriorates.

Nursing need not jump too readily on the RCT bandwagon. As was pointed out earlier, after much effort is expended in carrying out an RCT, the results can be disappointing (Tannock, 1992). Nevertheless, it is an important research method and, as a conference sponsored by the National Center for Nursing Research (1992b) (now National Institute of Nursing Research) concluded, it will likely play a larger role in nursing research in the future. Therefore, it is important for nurses to be familiar with the essential characteristics of the RCT while maintaining an awareness of its limitations.

Chapter 7

Outcome Measures

Introduction

Outcome measures play an important role in both research and practice. The measurement of outcomes evaluates the efficacy of interventions: the extent to which a medication, procedure, or program produced a desired effect. Outcomes measurement is not only useful in research on therapeutic interventions, but in research in which interventions are diagnostic, preventive, or rehabilitative. Outcome measures are also important in quality assurance programs that evaluate whether care delivered adheres to certain criteria or standards.

The importance of outcome measures in nursing has been underscored by the publication of a four-volume compendium of measures of nursing outcomes (Strickland & Waltz, 1988, 1990; Waltz and Strickland, 1988, 1990). Included are outcome measures not only for clinical research, but also for research on nursing practice and nursing education. Another indication of the growing interest in outcome measures was a conference sponsored by the National Center for Nursing Research (now National Institute of Nursing Research) in 1991. The proceedings contain a number of papers on outcome measurement and data sources (National Center for Nursing Research, 1992b).

Also, in 1993, the Springer Publishing Company initiated a new journal, *Journal of Nursing Measurement*, devoted to measurement issues in nursing research.

Since its early history, outcome has been central to health care. Physicians and nurses have always been attuned to the results of clinical interventions. Has the patient gotten better? Has the fever gone down? Is one able to feed oneself without assistance? These are some of the questions that have been asked since the beginnings of nursing.

The measurement of outcomes in research, and especially clinical research, has received considerable attention as the rapid rise in costs of health care has stimulated the search for more cost-effective ways of delivering care. The federal government's Medical Treatment Effectiveness Program (MEDTEP) of the United States Public Health Service's Agency for Health Care Policy and Research was specifically mandated in 1989 to promote improved outcomes from treatments and procedures (Agency for Health Care Policy and Research [AHCPR], 1992).

The concept of health outcomes can be viewed within the context of a social interaction resulting from the relationship between the provider and recipient of a service. In the clinical setting a nurse performs a procedure with the expectation that it will result in a desirable outcome. Thus, there is a social relationship between the intervention by the nurse and the outcome in the patient. The social aspect complicates the measurement of outcomes because of the many confounding variables present in a social setting. Consequently, the search for valid, sensitive, and meaningful outcome measures in nursing is most challenging.

It is especially important in clinical research and in monitoring of patient progress that the outcome measure has clinical relevance. That is: there should be a logical and relevant connection between intervention and expected outcome. Moreover, the outcome measure must be sensitive to the intervention (Stewart & Archbold, 1993). This means that the measure should be refined enough to detect meaningful responses to the intervention.

Historical Development

Nurses and other caregivers have always used outcome measures in monitoring responses to care. Early measures were, for the most part, informal, nonquantitative, and subjective. Florence Nightingale's writings contain numerous references to the effects of nursing care. Accurate quantitative assessment of outcomes was made possible in the last century by the development of scientific instruments for the measurement of physiologic and other clinical variables. The establishment in 1883 of an internationally accepted classification of diseases provided the mechanism for using morbidity and mortality data as outcome measures (Levine & Abdellah, 1984).

Substantial interest in the formal development of outcome measures for research began in the late 1950s. One important stimulant was the federal government's support for nursing research, originated in 1955 (Abdellah & Levine, 1986). As a result, formal evaluations of nursing were initiated that required indicators of the outcomes of care. In a journal article that called attention to the importance of investigating the end results of nursing interventions, these indicators were designated *criterion measures* (Abdellah, 1961).

One of the earliest conceptualizations of the relationship between nursing care and patient outcomes described a number of measures of *patient welfare* that could be used to evaluate the effects of nursing (Aydelotte & Tener, 1960). These included number of days hospitalized after surgery, number of days the patient had a fever, and medications received. Other nursing studies conducted at this time introduced the concept of quantifying outcome variables through the use of scaling techniques (Howland & McDowell, 1964; Simon, 1961).

It is fair to say that nursing has been a leader in the health care field in the conceptual and methodological development of outcome measures for use in research. A two-volume publication, prepared by Ward and Lindeman (1978) for the Western Interstate Commission on Higher Education in Nursing (WICHEN), compiled a large variety of instruments for measuring nursing practice. A number of client-focused instruments were specifically identified as measures of outcomes for use in quality assurance programs. The previously cited four-volume work, published by the Springer Publishing Company in 1988 and 1990, contains instruments that measure nursing outcomes for use in research as well as in quality assurance programs.

Development of outcome measures in health was significantly expanded in the 1970s. A major effort at that time was a study to evaluate medical care outcomes (Brook et al., 1977). Interest in outcome measurement was stimulated by the following:

- Adoption of health planning legislation that attempted to rationalize the organization and delivery of health care;
- Initiation of efforts to contain escalating costs of health care by enhancing the efficacy and cost-effectiveness of medical interventions;

- Application of evaluation research to assess the accomplishments of health care programs;
- Use of clinical trials to evaluate the efficacy of drugs and other therapies; and
- Emphasis on the assessment of the quality of care through the use of outcome measures.

In the 1980s, cost containment methodologies such as diagnosis-related groups (DRGs) were pursued in efforts to contain health care costs. Interest in methodology to measure outcomes and quality of care appeared to wane, only to be revived in the 1990s with the proliferation of clinical trials, the initiation of the MEDTEP program and its work on clinical practice guidelines, and an increasing emphasis on health promotion and disease prevention programs.

Types of Outcome Measures

The variety of outcome measures is limitless, since almost any variable has the potential of being one. Take "hair color" as an example. This is a simple descriptive variable that could serve as an outcome measure in an evaluation of the effectiveness of hair color dyes. It could be "measured" subjectively by a rater using a simple nominal scale, or objectively and quantitatively using spectroscopic measurement.

Outcome measures can be classified according to the following typology:

Purpose of Use

There are at least three uses of outcome measures: measuring dependent variables in explanatory research; measuring quality of care for quality assurance programs; and monitoring a client's disease process or health status. The same outcome measure can be used for different purposes. For example, a functional assessment measure, such as *Activities of Daily Living* (ADL), can be used to evaluate early discharge of patients from hospital to a home care program. It can also be used in a quality assurance program for a nursing home or a home health agency to assess the performance of the nursing staff in accomplishing care goals. Finally, it can be used to monitor a person's clinical status in response to treatment.

Subject Focus

An outcome measure can be used to study people, animals, plants, minerals, human organizations, the programs, policies and procedures of organizations, or any other class of subjects that the human mind can conceive. An outcome measure can also be applied to individuals or to groups of individuals aggregated to whatever level is desired, e.g., a single patient care unit in a hospital, the whole hospital, all the hospitals in a state, or all the hospitals in the nation.

Subject Matter Focus

Depending on the purpose of its use, an outcome measure in which study subjects are people can address either physical, psychological, behavioral, educational, economic, or social characteristics. It can also be a composite of various characteristics. Outcome measures for organizations can focus on performance variables such as economic indicators, utilization measures, personnel turnover, and client satisfaction.

Unitary or Multidimensional

Some outcome measures are simple: unidimensional, homogeneous variables such as body temperature, blood pressure, frequency of bed sores, letters of complaint received, annual earnings, absenteeism, or job changes. Or they can be multidimensional, such as health status and quality of life indexes, which combine several variables into a comprehensive measure.

Instrument or Database

Data on some outcome measures are available from secondary sources. Data on physiologic and diagnostic measures may be available from existing databases such as client, insurance, or vital statistics records, and the like. Computerized data systems simplify retrieval of this information, assuming protection of confidentiality is ensured. Even multidimensional measures can be constructed from these data bases. A researcher should resort to instrument development and collection of primary data only when there are no usable databases. If it is necessary to collect primary data, the instrument does not have to be tailor-made for the study, but may be selected from existing instruments.

Objective or Subjective

Measures of outcome can be obtained in many different ways, ranging from objective quantitative readings of scientific scales to subjective observations of qualitative phenomena. Qualitative methodology can be used to obtain information about phenomena that can help develop outcome measures.

Scale of Measurement

Measurement scales for outcome measures include nominal scales as in a disease classification; ordinal scales as in a functional capability scale; and the quantitative scales—both interval and ratio—used in clinical measurements.

Direct or Indirect

Outcome measures need not necessarily be literally defined, because it may be impossible to obtain a direct measurement of the outcome. Indirect measures can be meaningful and accurate indicators of outcomes, sometimes even more meaningful than direct measures. For example, how is the variable "quality of life" (QOL) measured directly? It may be possible to construct a psychosocial instrument that provides a score based on a battery of questions. Alternatively, certain behaviors could be measured that are indicative of QOL. Does the subject attend social functions? Read books? Attend concerts? Travel?

Another approach, quite indirect, is a content analysis of a person's verbal behavior obtained from recordings. Instruments are available that purport to provide a personality profile based on an analysis of a person's everyday conversation, handwriting, or body language.

Short or Long Run

Depending on the specific context in which the outcome measure is being used, the measurement may be made over the short or long run. Presence or absence of a simple headache to test the efficacy of various kinds of pain killers can be measured over a brief time span, in hours or even minutes. The efficacy of treatment for migraine headaches may require outcome measurement over a longer period, for months at least. The efficacy of dietary changes on longevity could take a lifetime to assess.

Prospective or Retrospective

Outcome measures can be used prospectively or retrospectively. A clear example of prospective use is the randomized clinical trial, where intervention precedes measurement of outcomes. In retrospective studies, such as epidemiological studies, the outcome is observed and then linked to the intervention or causal factor. Nursing evaluation studies frequently use the retrospective approach. For example, a high incidence of pressure sores is observed. The extent to which they are related to such causal factors as decreased mobility, devitalized state of health, age, and medical diagnosis is then investigated. Recent studies of risk factors associated with major illnesses such as lung cancer, breast cancer, and cardiovascular disease began with observation of high death rates from these diseases, which were later traced back to such practices as heavy cigarette smoking and fatty diets.

New or Borrowed Measures

A prospective study can design a new outcome measure or use an existing one. The WICHEN and Springer books have provided a fine service for researchers by bringing together in one place a diverse collection of outcome measures. Journals are also a good source of outcome measures and data collection instruments. Retrospective studies use existing outcome measures based on secondary data. However, it is possible to construct new outcome measures from secondary data, as is done in meta-analyses.

A researcher embarking on a new study can develop an outcome measure from scratch, which may require considerable effort, or use one "off the shelf." The temptation may be to design a new measure. Because this can consume many resources, it is cost-efficient to use an existing measuring instrument whenever possible, particularly a well-tested one. An existing instrument can be modified, if necessary, to fit a new study.

Assessment of Outcome Measures

The quality of outcome measures is assessed by the same criteria used to evaluate the adequacy, sufficiency, and efficiency of measurement generally. Are the measures free of errors? Are they meaningful as relevant indicators of the outcomes of the interventions being evaluated? Are they easy to use and interpret (Perlow, 1988)? The criteria include:

Validity

This criterion assesses whether the outcome measure actually measures what it is supposed to measure. For example, if the measure is of a person's functional capability, does it accurately assess this variable? Do differences in scales to measure the variable reflect real differences in functional capability?

Reliability

This refers to the consistency and stability of the measure. A measure is reliable if it is consistently reproducible. That is, independent measurements of a person's functional capability, taken within the same period, should yield the same results. Reliability is less important than validity, because a measure that is consistently inaccurate is useless.

Sensitivity

The sensitivity criterion assesses the capability of the measure to detect fine differences among study subjects. Sensitivity depends on the scale of measurement. Crude scales with only a few qualitative categories are less sensitive than finely graded quantitative scales. A scale with only two categories, such as functionally capable or incapable, is less sensitive than one that has many categories.

Meaningfulness

This criterion assesses the outcome measure pragmatically. It questions whether or not the measure has relevance. A measure used as an indicator of outcomes is meaningful if it can influence decisions and actions relating to the delivery of care. Thus, for example, if a functional capability measure is meaningful it should, in a study of the effects of early discharge of elderly hospital patients, yield information that can help make decisions about need for care after discharge.

The criterion of meaningfulness bears a relationship to the construct validity of a measure, referring not only to the validity of the measure itself, but to the validity of the underlying theory (Selltiz, Wrightsman, & Cook, 1976). The criterion is similar to the concept of practical significance of research findings; that is, the extent to which the findings can be consistently and realistically applied. The validity of a measure does not guarantee that it is meaningful, although, of course, an invalid or unreliable measure would be meaningless.

The remainder of this chapter will discuss two categories of outcome measures that are particularly relevant to nursing research: measures of health status and measures of *nursing* outcomes.

Measures of Health Status

The concept of a person's health can be defined in a number of ways. The World Health Organization (WHO) in a 1978 report on primary health care defined health as a state of complete physical, mental, and social well-being (World Health Organization [WHO], 1978). In 1984 WHO presented a set of health status indicators that would measure this holistic definition of health (WHO, 1984).

A more restricted definition of health is simply "absence of disease." Still another introduces the concept of *level of wellness*, which, like the WHO definition, is focused on health, not disease (Dunn, 1959). Newman (1991) offers a conceptualization in terms of a wellness-illness continuum.

These definitions leave something to be desired as the basis for developing outcome measures for nursing research. While the WHO definition is inclusive, it is difficult to operationalize and quantify, and somewhat utopian. Health as absence of disease, based on the illness-oriented medical model, is a limited conception of health status because a person can have a medically defined disease, yet lead an active and productive life.

Outcome measures of health include a wide range of variables, sometimes called the "five d's:" dissatisfaction, discomfort, disability, disease, and death (White, 1974). These are all negative criteria, while the emphasis on wellness needs positive outcomes such as giving up smoking, eating less fatty food, exercising, and other beneficial life-style changes.

Most studies do not attempt to measure health globally. In a research study the measurement of health status outcomes may focus on a single characteristic such as presence or absence of a disease, condition, symptom, health problem, or health behavior. These are *unidimensional measures of health status*. More comprehensive measures of health status combine several variables. Known as *health indexes or health profiles*, multidimensional measures of health status can include psychosocial and behavioral variables as well as physical ones. Concepts of level of wellness and quality of life usually include all of these variables.

The concept of health, from both the illness and wellness perspectives, is becoming increasingly important in nursing research. One reason is the clinical orientation of many recent nursing studies. Also, the development of nursing theories and models has stimulated the conceptualization and definition of health. Another factor has been the growing interest in testing nursing interventions for the promotion of health and prevention of disease. Health status measures are quite important in evaluating outcomes of wellness programs. The objectives of the federal government for improving the health of Americans by the year 2000 through health promotion and disease prevention programs are formulated in terms of health status outcome measures (McGinnis, Richmond, Brandt, Windom, & Mason, 1992; U. S. Department of Health and Human Services, 1991).

Health status measures are of interest not only to researchers and clinicians, but to health policy analysts. The term *health indicator* describes a health status measure that has relevance for developing and monitoring health policies. The infant mortality rate is an example of an indicator used in international comparisons to assess the effectiveness of a nation's health system. The recent trend in the use of health status indicators has been towards evaluation of policy-relevant issues.

Historical Roots of Health Status Measures

The measurement of health status has had a long and eventful history. It began with a focus on disease, which is understandable since, until recently, health care consisted primarily of the diagnosis and treatment of sickness.

The first step in the measurement of health status was development of a classification scale for diseases. The origin of disease classification—descriptions of human pathology—are found in the Old Testament, Egyptian medical treatises from about 3000 BC, and ancient Chinese texts. In the fifth century BC, Hippocrates developed a rudimentary classification of diseases. Further developed by Galen in the second century AD, these classifications greatly influenced "medical" practice, for the most part negatively, until well past the Middle Ages.

Early categorizations of diseases were used diagnostically by physicians to determine the appropriate course of treatment for a patient. The use of a disease classification for *epidemiological* evaluations was undertaken in London in 1662 by John Graunt who had been directed by the king to analyze the causes of death contributing to the 40% mortality rate in children under 6 years of age. Two hundred years later, in 1853, the British statistician William Farr organized the first International Statistical Congress in Brussels in which the idea of a standard international classification of diseases was discussed.

In 1891 Jacques Bertillon chaired a committee of the International Statistical Institute that produced the International Classification of Diseases (ICD). Officially adopted in 1893, this has become the standard taxonomy for classifying and reporting data on causes of death (mortality) and sickness (morbidity). Periodically revised and updated, the ICD is now in its tenth revision. The classification contains over 10,000 categories in its "scale."

Mortality and Morbidity Data

Mortality Data

The ICD is widely used throughout the world to report causes of death from the death certificates required to be filed by physicians. The immediate cause of death is reported as well as underlying causes, if any. In the United States, death certificates are processed through the National Vital Statistics System of the federal government. Annual statistics are published on causes of death by age, sex, ethnicity, and geographic location. These data are useful in epidemiologic studies of large populations. Death and sickness rates are also used as outcome measures in randomized clinical trials.

Mortality data provide a narrow view of health status. In assessing population groups, reductions in mortality rates do not necessarily mean that health status has been improved. Fewer people may be dying but more people may be sick, disabled, depressed, or dysfunctional. Mortality data reveal nothing about quality of life and have only a limited use as outcome measures in nursing research. The objectives of nursing interventions include reduction of disability and discomfort and improvement of quality of life. Pertinent health outcomes for nursing are wellness-oriented, not death- or disease-oriented.

When used as outcome measures mortality data are expressed as rates: in terms of the number of deaths per unit of population. Because the number of deaths is usually quite small in relation to size of population, the mortality rate is expressed in terms of number of deaths per population unit that varies from 100 to 100,000 persons and allows the rate to be stated in whole numbers. The mortality rate for deaths from all causes for the United States is computed in terms of units of 100,000 persons. For smaller populations such as study groups in clinical trials, the population units can be per 100 or 1,000.

In 1989 the *crude death rate* for all causes of death in the United States was 866 deaths per 100,000 population (United States Department of Health and Human Services, 1992). Because the age composition of the population changes each year, an *age-adjusted death rate* is calculated by weighting the deaths occurring in each age group by a standard age distribution. The age-adjusted death rate is important in comparing geographic areas such as states or countries where peoples' ages differ. In 1989 the age-adjusted death rate for the U.S. was 523 per 100,000 population (or 5 per 1,000).

In addition to adjusting for age distribution of the population, various other refinements can be made to the crude death rate to make it more meaningful as an outcome measure. One interesting measure is called the *years of potential life lost* (YPLL). This is calculated as follows: for each death the difference between actual age at death and expected age according to estimates of life expectancy is computed. Thus, if a death occurs in a white male at age 66 and the life expectancy for white males is 72, the YPLL is 6. The YPLL for deaths among white males 72 and over is zero. To calculate the YPLL *rate*, the differences between actual and expected ages for all deaths are added, divided by the total population, and multiplied by 100,000. The YPLL rate for specific diseases is especially informative. As expected, the YPLL for AIDS is very high.

Morbidity

The ICD is used to classify diseases as well as causes of death, although reporting of diseases, except for certain communicable diseases, is not legally required. Since World War II there has been increasing interest in gathering data on the incidence and prevalence of noncommunicable diseases. Several ongoing sample surveys conducted by the federal government's National Center for Health Statistics provide considerable data on illnesses, injuries, impairments, and chronic conditions, published annually for large population groups (U. S. Department of Health and Human Services, 1992). The most comprehensive of these is the *National Health Interview Study*. The *National Hospital Discharge Survey* provides diagnostic data on a sample of patients discharged from short-stay hospitals. Another source of data on morbidity are the databases for Medicare patients maintained by the federal government's Health Care Financing Administration (HCFA).

As outcome measures, morbidity data suffer from the same shortcoming as do mortality data: insensitivity. A strictly nominal measure, it states that the person either does or does not have the disease, but gives no indication of its severity or its impact on a person's life. Moreover, medical diagnoses of the ICD do not give information on the nursing problems and interventions associated with the diagnosis.

Two variants of morbidity data have increased their meaningfulness as health status measures: the problem-oriented record and nursing diagnoses. These methodologies, designed for use in the planning and delivery of care, are also useful as outcome measures.

The Problem-Oriented Reporting System

Although Lawrence Weed is credited with originating the problem-oriented medical record (POMR) in the 1960s, the problem approach to describing deviations from health can be found in the nursing literature which predates Weed by many years (Hanchett, 1977; Weed, 1964). Florence Nightingale refers to patients' problems that should be attended by nurses. The 1934 study of the Committee on the Grading of Nursing Schools transformed medical diagnoses into activities (problems) that are the responsibilities of nurses (Johns & Pfefferkorn, 1934). Nursing care planning based on a conceptualization of patient problems was described in Harmer's and Henderson's revision of their classic textbook (1939). Fry (1953) identified five areas of patients' problems that could serve as a basis for nursing diagnosis. Abdellah (1957) described a patient-centered approach to determining nursing problems. In 1961 she showed how problems could be used as outcome measures to assess goal attainment in the nursing process.

Weed's problem-oriented system has four components: database, problem list, initial plans, and progress notes. The POMR replaces the conventional patient record and expands the reporting of medical diagnoses based on the ICD taxonomy by describing them in terms of the health problems addressable by medical and nursing providers, thus creating a process for care planning and progress monitoring.

Problem-oriented reporting overcomes the limitations of a diagnosis based on a disease classification that gives little information on the actual health status and needs of the person. For example, two people may have the same disease classification, yet have very different health problems requiring different interventions. A person with myocardial infarction may exhibit a number of problems such as pain, weakness, and anxiety, while another person with the same diagnosis may have a different set of problems or exhibit no problems at all. Problem-oriented reporting provides information about the intervention needed; the medical diagnosis does not.

The problem-oriented system was primarily designed to improve delivery of clinical care. It was also believed to be useful as a method for auditing care and to provide a meaningful framework for educating physicians and other providers by replacing static diagnoses with active descriptors of deviations from health.

Initially, the use of a problem list to generate outcome measures in research was not viewed as feasible because the classification scale is only nominal. However, even nominal scales are useful as outcome measures. A comparison can be made of a person's problems before and after the intervention. The problems observed after care can be analyzed as indicators of the effects of intervention.

Nursing Diagnoses

Nursing diagnoses, discussed by Harmer and Henderson (1939), Fry (1953), Abdellah (1957, 1961) and others years ago, were popularized in the 1970s along with the concept of *nursing process*. The nursing process was defined as consisting of five components: assessment, analysis, planning, implementation, and evaluation (Atkinson & Murray, 1983; Yura & Walsh, 1978). Nursing diagnoses play an important role in this framework, primarily in the functions of assessing, planning, and evaluating.

The North American Nursing Diagnosis Association (NANDA) developed a standardized list of diagnoses based on problem orientation. Examples include ineffective airway clearance, impairment of skin integrity, and sleep pattern disturbance.

In 1985 a conference was held to identify the nursing minimum data set (Werley & Lang, 1988). Six task forces, grouped according to the components of the nursing process, were established to identify the most essential items of information required to provide nursing care. One task force was charged with determining how data should be organized and collected in the measurement of nursing diagnoses. It defined a nursing diagnosis as a clinical judgement about a human response to an actual or potential health problem for which nursing is accountable and recommended that the NANDA list of diagnoses be used in the nursing minimum dataset.

As outcome measures, nursing diagnoses have the same limitations as do POMR problems. They are unscaled and provide a rudimentary nominal "measure." In addition, diagnoses, since they largely describe deviations from health, seem somewhat anachronistic in the current "wellness" climate.

Other Measures of General Health Status

In addition to problems and diagnoses there is a large amount of health-status related data existing in databases. Included are counts of days a person was hospitalized, days of absenteeism, restricted activity days, symptoms and signs, impairments, and laboratory test results. In addition, there are paper-and-pencil instruments that can be used to obtain a person's self-rating of health status as well as ratings by physicians and nurses. The *Cornell Medical Index* (1951) is a comprehensive self-evaluation instrument that contains about 200 "yes-no" questions pertaining to frequency of illness, lifestyle, mood, and physiological problems. More recent instruments, such as the *Health Perceptions Questionnaire*, have refined the Cornell Index, but like other similar self-administered instruments they measure feelings and perceptions about health and not health status (Kane & Kane, 1981; Ware, 1976).

Scaled Measures of Dependency and Functional Status

Functional status is an important indicator of health status. In the most comprehensive sense, functional status measures the adequacy of a person's physical, mental, and social performance. Functional status, which can be quantified in an ordinal scale, is a more relevant indicator of health status than is an unweighted list of diseases, symptoms, signs, or impairments.

The history of the development of functional status measures again reveals the important role of nursing, although one of the first attempts to scale health was oriented to medical care. Roger Lee and Barbara Jones in the early 1930s estimated the number of physicians required to serve the nation's medical needs (Lee & Jones, 1933). Using the 1920 revision of the ICD they determined the incidence of major illnesses. They then calculated the number of physician hours required to treat these illnesses, a process of weighting (scaling) the diagnostic categories by physician requirements. This procedure was followed 50 years later by the development of diagnosis related groups (DRGs) (Levine & Abdellah, 1984).

Patient Classification for Nursing Management

In 1934 the nurses Ethel Johns and Blanche Pfefferkorn published their classic study,*An Activity Analysis of Nursing*, for the Committee on the Grading of Nursing Schools, in which they developed a list of conditions that required nursing interventions. These conditions included not only curative and therapeutic interventions for ill persons, but preventive measures as well.

The National League for Nursing Education (NLNE) then sponsored a series of studies that led to development of what is known today as patient classification scales (Giovannetti, 1978; National League for Nursing Education [NLNE] 1937, 1947, 1948). One of the earliest scales of this type was reported by the NLNE in 1947 in a study of needs for pediatric nurses. It assessed four patient factors: degree of illness (acute, moderate, long-term), extent of activity, number and complexity of treatments and procedures, and nature of behavioral adjustment. This scale possessed the theoretical framework of contemporary health status indexes and functional status measures.

Basically, patient classification scales classify patients according to their needs for or dependency on nursing care. They are used to determine nursing requirements. Literally hundreds of such scales exist today. Most are applicable to patients in acute care hospitals, but there are scales for patients in psychiatric hospitals, nursing homes, and home care. These instruments differ in scale refinement, varying from unweighted nominal scales to fully quantified scales. Some scales are part of elaborate patient classification systems that include assessment instruments, computerized processing, and care planning methodology (Giovannetti & Thiessen, 1983).

Although these scales are mainly used for resource management, they can also be used to measure outcomes. Their drawback as a measure of health status is that they concentrate on attributes for which nursing interventions are applicable. Therefore, they are only partial health status measures. Their main use has been in hospitals and nursing homes. However, even with these limitations they can be useful in assessing changes in dependency status (O'Brien-Pallas, Cockerill, & Leatt, 1992).

Comprehensive Functional Assessment

The development of functional status measures was stimulated by federal legislation: Medicare (1965), Comprehensive Health Planning (1966), and the Health Planning and Resources Development Act (1975). Medicare greatly expanded costs of health care. The health planning programs, now largely defunct, were an attempt to control costs through rational management of resources. Assessment of functional status, particularly the status of geriatric patients, had several purposes, a major one being to increase cost-effective utilization of health resources by determining whether a patient should be cared for in a hospital, nursing home, or at home.

The most widely known functional assessment scale, the Activities of Daily Living (ADL), was first described by Katz and others in 1963 (Katz, Ford, Moskowitz, Jackson, & Jaffee, 1963). The ADL scale is similar to previously discussed *nursing* patient classification scales developed in the 1950s, which, in turn, had antecedents in the earlier work of Johns, Pfefferkorn, Rovetta, Bredenburg, and others (Bredenburg, 1951; Johns & Pfefferkorn, 1934; Pfefferkorn, 1932; Pfefferkorn & Rovetta, 1940). The Katz ADL scale rates the capability of a person to perform six tasks: bathing, dressing, going to toilet, transferring, controlling continence, and feeding. Each task is scaled according to the degree of independent functioning of the person and an aggregate score obtained for the six tasks. Originally the scale for each task was dichotomous, but refinements introduced Guttman-type scales,

ADL scales have been used for a variety of purposes including outcome measures in research on nursing interventions. Although used mainly with older people, the measurement of ADL is applicable to all ages. The popularity of these scales lies in their ease of use and their validity and reliability.

In the late 1960s refinements to the ADL scale began to be made. Although the emphasis was still on physical functioning, new dimensions were added. Lawton and Brody (1969) introduced the *Instrumental Activities of Daily Living* (IADL) scale. The IADL measures performance on eight everyday tasks such as using the telephone, preparing meals, shopping, and managing money. These are more complex than ADL functions and, to a certain extent, have a mental as well as physical component.

Other extensions of the ADL, such as the *Patient Classification for Long Term Care*, included additional functions (stair-climbing), refined the scales into a larger number of categories, and added measures of impairments to the instrument (Jones, 1974). The *Older American's Resources and Services Inventory* (OARS) developed at Duke University is a multidimensional functional assessment instrument combining ADL, IADL, and social and mental status items (Duke University Center for the Study of Aging, 1978). As part of a major study of health insurance conducted in the 1970s, the Rand Corporation produced a functional assessment instrument that included a 13-item functional limitations battery and a 12-item physical capacities battery that measured performance in lifting, walking, and engaging in athletics (Stewart, Ware, & Brook, 1982). The study defined functional status as the performance of or the capacity to perform a variety of activities normal for a person in good health.

Thus, the trend has been from a limited measure of functional status that assesses basic physical capabilities and performance to a more comprehensive measure that includes complex physical functions, as well as the mental, behavioral, and social components of functional capacity (Kane & Kane, 1981; Lohr, 1989, 1992). The newer measures are oriented more to accomplishments and capabilities than to limitations. As the measures have become more multidimensional, they have acquired the characteristics of a global index of health status. A global index, like economic indices that measure the gross national product and cost of living, has many important uses including health policy formulation, health planning, resources management, and outcome measures in research.

Quality of Life

One health status measure to which increasing attention is being paid is *Quality of Life* (QOL) (Murdagh, 1992). For the most part, the measurement of QOL, like the measurement of functional status, has been applied to elderly people with chronic and disabling health problems. This measurement is important for several reasons. First, there is the growing awareness that the reality of "being alive" can vary, from a totally incapacitated person living on a respirator to a productive person who is functioning with high levels of physical, social, and psychic energy. Second, if a valid and reliable measure of QOL could be designed, it would have many valuable uses as a measure of outcome in evaluation research. Third, the current emphasis on health promotion and disease prevention activities increases the need for measures of the qualitative aspect of a person's life. How often does one hear that "If I have to give up smoking, or drinking, or eating good food, my life is not worth living." The attitude is that there is more to the meaning and value of life than duration alone. In short, there is interaction among the concepts of quality of life, health status, and outcomes.

At this time there is no widely accepted measure of QOL, like the ADL, nor is there agreement on its definition. Early scales viewed the quality of life in terms of a life free of disability or illness and measured it by combining mortality and morbidity rates into a single index (Chiang, 1965; Sullivan, 1966). Later definitions include two dimensions: functioning and perceptions (Wenger, Mattson, Furberg, & Elinson, 1984). The current view appears to be that the concept of QOL is multifactorial and includes a variety of subjective and objective measures. It is also likely that repeated measurements of the QOL of the same individual will show considerable variation over time (Spilker, 1986).

Lawton has provided an interesting framework for assessing QOL (Lawton, 1982, 1987). He describes four overlapping sectors of the good life: psychological well-being, behavioral competence, objective environment, and perceived quality of life. Psychological well-being refers to general mental health, absence of depression, positive affect, and so on. Behavior competence includes ADLs, IADLs, and adequacy of a person's social behavior. The objective environment is composed of variables such as housing quality, population density, and social network. Perceived quality of life relates to a subjective evaluation of quality of behavior. Thus, a QOL index can be constructed that combines measurements of the four dimensions.

It is clear that there are many health status measures that could be used as outcome measures in nursing research. Most are generic measures and, except for patient classification scales and nursing diagnoses, do not specifically relate to nursing interventions. However, these measures do have a high degree of relevance in studies where the desired outcome is improvement in health status.

Outcome Measures Specific to Nursing

A final category of outcome measures is those that have been customized for nursing studies. A number of these measures and the instruments for collecting the data are included in the previously cited compilations (Waltz & Strickland, 1988; Ward & Lindeman, 1978). In addition, a literature search should uncover many instruments and measures from research reports and journal articles. A review of these measures reveals much variety in content and methodology.

Nursing-specific outcome measures can be divided into three main categories according to the object of measurement: clients who receive nursing services, the services provided, and the environment in which the services are provided. Interestingly, this classification is similar to the quality-of-care paradigm: *outcomes* in terms of recipients of services, *process* in terms of providers of services, and *structure* in terms of setting and resources in which services are provided. It is necessary to keep in mind, however, that outcome measurement and measurement of the quality of care are not the same thing. Outcome measures are used in quality-of-care assessments, but they are also used for other purposes such as clinical monitoring of patients and testing therapeutic interventions.

Outcome measures can also be used to evaluate the efficacy and effectiveness of the process and structure domains. A study of the effect of continuing education on nursing performance is an example of an evaluation in which changes in process are the measured outcomes. Similarly, quality-of-care assessments can utilize outcome criteria relating to process and structure as well as criteria relating to recipients of care. In nursing, outcome measurement is used more often in assessing quality of care than in research. This is likely to change in the future as more clinical studies, including clinical trials, are undertaken to evaluate nursing interventions.

Client-Focused Outcome Measures

These can include the whole array of health status measures and indicators previously discussed, including measures of functional capabilities and sociopsychological and behavioral variables. Examples can also be cited of health status measures expressly designed for nursing applications, such as the various patient classification instruments.

One example of a nursing-developed, client-focused outcome measure is an instrument to assess the status at discharge of patients hospitalized with myocardial infarction (Haussmann & Hegyvary, 1977). The instrument was designed as part of a major project to develop methodology to measure the quality of nursing care (Jelinek, Haussmann, Hegyvary, & Newman, 1974). It is a multidimensional index consisting of eight scales: general health status, rest and sleep, ADL, general health knowledge, medication knowledge, activity knowledge, nutrition knowledge, and anxiety.

Other nursing outcome measures have ranged from focus on specific physical problems such as pain, pressure sores, and airway obstruction, to psychological and behavioral problems such as compliance, anxiety, and depression, and to wellness-oriented measures such as self-care capabilities, lifestyle, social interaction, and positive health beliefs (Waltz & Strickland, 1988; Ward & Lindeman, 1978). Outcome measures have been designed to address not only the primary recipient of services, but family members and the entire support system as well. Moreover, there are measures for every major health care setting including hospitals, nursing homes, and home care.

Patient Satisfaction

This nursing-oriented outcome measure has been receiving increased attention. As an indicator of either efficacy or quality of services, it has had many detractors as well as supporters. Consumers of care are not believed to be knowledgeable health care evaluators, since their judgments can be biased by prior experiences, extent of knowledge of health care, health status, and severity of health problems. Nevertheless, as a short-range response variable, patient satisfaction can be useful in evaluation research if interpreted carefully.

The measurement of patient satisfaction is another example of a research methodology originated by nurses. Prior to this century, nurses used simple, unscaled checklists to elicit patients' opinions about their hospital stay. In 1957 Abdellah and Levine designed a 52-item checklist for patients in acute care hospitals to report on various events related to their care. Items were grouped into seven categories such as rest and relaxation, dietary needs, and elimination. A similar checklist was designed for personnel. The checklists were scored by 9,000 patients and an equal number of personnel in 60 randomly selected hospitals and used as outcome measures to evaluate different nurse staffing patterns. Subsequent satisfaction scales were developed for other settings and for other responders including family members. Interest in patient satisfaction instruments was further stimulated by the *consumerism in health* movement of the 1970s which resulted in the *Patient's Bill of Rights*. Recent evaluations of consumer satisfaction with health care have targeted physicians and other health care providers.

Provider and Organization-Focused Outcome Measures

Many nursing interventions have been tested in which the outcomes of interest are the effects on nursing staff or the work setting. These include studies of nursing performance, creativity, education, professional development, and stability. Also included are studies of nursing organizational performance, resources, and stability. An example is an instrument—actually a collection of tests—to evaluate the clinical performance of critical care nurses (Mims, 1988). Five areas of performance were conceptualized: assessment, clinical/technical skill, communication, documentation, and general employment policies. Twenty-four separate tests were designed to rate performance in these five areas. Although primarily designed to be used as a management tool, this instrument can also be used to evaluate educational programs, leadership styles, work incentives, and so forth.

Use of Outcome Measures in Nursing

Much effort has been expended in developing outcome measures for nursing research. These measures can be used in other studies as long as they are relevant and the measuring instrument is valid and reliable. Just as the use of secondary data can be a cost-effective way of conducting a study, so can the use of existing methodology.

The criteria of relevance and validity are extremely important in the selection of an outcome measure for a study, whether an existing measure is used or a new one is developed. Consider that what may seem to be a perfectly sound outcome measure of health status, such as mortality or morbidity, may be inappropriate for nursing. Because a patient has a course of illness in which death is inevitable, regardless of the nursing interventions provided, mortality is thus a poor indicator for most nursing studies. Morbidity is also a weak measure for nursing research; the problem-oriented nursing diagnosis is better. For many nursing studies another focus is needed, one that relates nursing care to outcomes in a meaningful way. It is here that *quality of care* becomes an important indicator. The following chapter is devoted to an examination of this concept.

Chapter 8

Measuring The Quality of Care

Introduction

Concern about the quality of nursing care, a common theme in the writings of Florence Nightingale and other early nursing leaders, continues undiminished to this day. In recent years escalating costs of health care, coupled with deficiencies in many aspects of the health care system, have given strong impetus to the development of methodology for measuring and analyzing the quality of care (Walker, 1992). Quality of care and outcome measures have much in common. Quality of care can be defined and measured in terms of outcomes. Additionally, it can serve as an outcome measure in evaluations of nursing interventions.

To define quality of care requires a definition of the attributes of care as well as the criteria for what constitutes good care. Care activities can be divided into *technical* and *interpersonal* (Donabedian, 1988). Technical care is the application of the science and technology of nursing and other health sciences to the management of a health problem. Interpersonal activities include the sociopsychological aspects of the nurse/patient interaction.

The concept of quality of care implies adherence to a standard that describes the accepted way in which technical and interpersonal activities should be carried out. The question to be answered in the assessment of quality of care is, "Was the right thing done and was it done right?" (Wyszewianski, 1988). Thus, assessment of quality of care presupposes that standards exist to evaluate that the right thing was done and that it was done properly. By contrast, clinical trials measure the efficacy of interventions and aim to discover the right thing to do. The clinical trial does not presuppose a standard: it assists in establishing one.

The pursuit of quality measurement, thus, involves two stages. The first stage requires the determination of standards. According to the American Nurses' Association (1991), there are two types of standards necessary for nursing: *standards of care* and *standards of performance*. The Association defines standards of care as *authoritative* descriptions of the performance of *competent* clinical practice.

Standards usually denote above-average performance and may even address optimality. Standards can be determined from formal, prospective research such as clinical trials. They can also be determined from retrospective analysis of existing data, but may be considered only provisional until more definitive information becomes available. Standards can also be set by the clinical judgment of experts, although this process often leads to definition of *norms*—average practice—rather than to optimal standards.

The second stage in the pursuit of quality measurement is construction of quality assessment methodology that incorporates the standards or norms into an operational instrument. The objective of quality measurement is to compare actual to optimal performance, determining the extent to which one deviates from the other. Basically, then, measuring the quality of care can focus on whether the right thing was done (what was accomplished) or whether it was done right (how it was done), or, most desirably, on both, in a procedure that links performance to accomplishments. Research comes into the picture in determining standards and norms, developing of the assessment methodology, and carrying out studies involving quality of care issues.

Historical Evolution

Early Studies

One of the earliest studies of nursing to attempt to determine standards of care for nursing was an evaluation of the activities of nurses in hospitals, undertaken in 1926 under the auspices of the Committee on the Grading of Nursing Schools (Johns & Pfefferkorn, 1934). The basic research question for the study was: What is good nursing? More specifically, the study asked, "What should a professional nurse know and be able to do?" The study delineated in detail the activities of nurses in various settings. Although written 60 years ago the study report still has relevance today. One example: "Nurses themselves must have a share in determining what the standards of professional practice shall be, for it is they who must be depended upon to integrate and coordinate all levels of nursing service" (Johns & Pfefferkorn, 1934, p. 19). In 1932 one of the authors of the report discussed the need to evaluate the quality as well as the quantity of nursing care (Pfefferkorn, 1932).

The Johns and Pfefferkorn study ushered in a long series of research projects supported by the National League for Nursing Education to determine appropriate staffing patterns for the delivery of nursing care in hospitals (Abdellah & Levine, 1986). Focusing on the nursing process, the objective of the studies was to determine the appropriate quantity and mix of nursing personnel necessary to assure good care.

A number of projects were initiated in the 1950s that focused on the "goodness" of care as well as its quantitative aspects. A study reported at the beginning of the decade made a direct attempt to measure the quality of care provided in hospitals (O'Malley & Kossack, 1950). In a staffing study reported in 1951, Bredenberg measured the amount of time nurses spent on non-nursing clerical activities as a criterion of the quality of care. Another study attempted to delineate the criteria for the assessment of the quality of nursing care (Reiter & Kakosh, 1963).

Role Studies

There were also during this period a large number of studies, supported by the American Nurses Association and state associations, investigating the roles and functions of nurses (Hughes, Hughes, & Deutscher, 1958). Although these were not strictly studies of the quality of nursing care, they did provide useful normative data on the work of nurses. Similarly, the nursing activity studies conducted by the federal government's Division of Nursing Resources generated a considerable amount of useful descriptive data (U.S Department of Health, Education and Welfare, 1954).

126 • NURSING METHODOLOGIES

Methodology to Evaluate Quality of Care

Formal methodology to assess quality of care became available in the 1950s beginning with a method of auditing medical records (Lembcke, 1956). A project to design a nursing audit was also initiated based on the concept of the medical audit (Phaneuf, 1976).

Abdellah and Levine (1957) developed instruments to measure patient and personnel satisfaction. Although they were used as outcome measures in a study of nursing staffing patterns in hospitals, these instruments could also be used to evaluate quality of care. Another study undertaken in the 1950s examined the impact of the quantity and mix of nursing personnel on a large number of measures of patient welfare (Aydelotte & Tener, 1960). Both the concepts of patient satisfaction and patient welfare would later serve as outcome measures in both efficacy and quality of care studies.

The Quality Paradigm

A major contribution to quality of care measurement was Sheps' classification (1955) of different approaches to the evaluation of quality of hospital care. Methods for evaluating quality of care were grouped into four categories:

- Characteristics of the hospital;
- Performance of staff;
- Effects on patients; and
- Clinical evaluations.

These categories can be put into a framework similar to the *operations research* model formulated in the 1940s to measure productivity of workers in defense plants. This model, building on Frederick Taylor's principles of *scientific management*, defined productivity as the ratio of output to input, in which output is measured by the number of units produced at a standard level of quality and input is measured by employee hours expended in making the units (Shewhart, 1931). Input and output are, in turn, related to the environment in which work takes place (see Figure 8.1).

Management theorists, particularly those of the human relations and cybernetics schools, elaborated on this simple model. Input was viewed not only as number of hours of employee time, but as the interaction and feedback of a number of variables including organization of work, procedures and processes, setting, technology, and

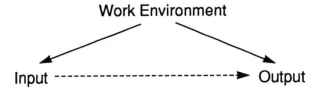

Figure 8.1   Input and output as they relate to the work environment.

interpersonal relationships. Improvements in productivity could be made by changes in any of these variables, especially, according to the theory of management known as human relations, in the key variables of leadership, teamwork, and employee participation in decision making. The concept of *Total Quality Management* (TQM) can be traced to the human relations theorists.

Donabedian (1966), to whom much credit is given for advancing the measurement of the quality of care, regrouped Sheps' (1955) categories into three interrelated concepts:

- Structure
- Process
- Outcome

Thus, the dynamic model becomes:

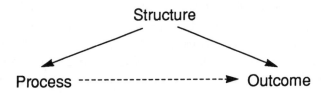

Figure 8.2. The three concepts of the dynamic model.

Each of these concepts includes a set of subvariables. Structure (which earlier management theorists labeled work environment) includes such variables as physical layout, fiscal and other resources, and technology. Process (the "input" of the operations research model) includes the content and flow of the work performed. Outcome is the end result of the work performed that can be measured by outcome measures.

Quality assessment can focus on any of the variables included in this model. Conventional wisdom has maintained that outcome provides the most meaningful measure of quality of care although, as will be discussed later, the outcome approach to quality assessment raises difficult issues.

Professional Service Review Organizations (PSROs)

Much activity occurred in the 1970s in measurement of quality of health care because of rapidly rising costs and increasing consumer dissatisfaction. In 1972 the Social Security Amendments mandated the Professional Standards Review Organization (PSRO) program to monitor the quality of all medical care services provided to individuals under Medicare, Medicaid, and Maternal and Child Health Programs of the federal government. The purpose was to determine whether services were medically necessary, met professionally recognized standards of care, and were cost-effective. Now known as the Professional Review Organization (PRO) program, this legislation was an important milestone in the development of quality assurance programs in all types of health care settings.

Measurement of the Quality of the Nursing Process

In the mid 1970s the federal government issued a series of publications describing a method for monitoring the quality of nursing care (Hegyvary & Haussmann, 1976; Jelinek, et al, 1974). The methodology was focused on measurement of performance (process) in hospitals. It consisted of a comprehensive set of 257 items, of which 205 were directed to patients and 52 to the nursing unit. Items were grouped into six categories representing the major objectives of the nursing process, and these were further subdivided into 28 subcategories. The major objectives were:

- Plan of nursing care is formulated;
- Physical needs of the patient are attended;
- Non-physical needs of the patient are attended;
- Achievement of nursing care objectives is evaluated;
- Unit procedures are followed for the protection of all patients; and
- Delivery of nursing care is facilitated by administrative and managerial services.

The items, called criteria, were formulated in terms of specifically worded questions about objectives and subobjectives. The following is an excerpt from the objective *the physical needs of the patient are attended*:

Subobjective. The patient is protected from accident and injury:

- Is the patient's identification bracelet worn on his wrist or leg as appropriate?
- Is the patient positioned for optimal body alignment?
- Is the IV needle adequately secured in place?
- Is the patient with special equipment, such as IVs or other tubing, taught precautions in getting out of bed?

Scoring of the instrument is quite simple. Each subobjective is assigned a weight by the hospital's advisory committee. Thus, weights vary from one hospital to another depending on the importance placed on the subobjective. Each specific item is answered by the evaluator in terms of a yes/no dichotomy. An aggregate quality score is obtained by adding up the number of items answered "yes" in a subobjective which is then multiplied by the weight of the subobjective. Similarly, a total score is obtained by summing up the subobjective scores.

A number of other measures of nursing performance were produced in the 1970s. The Quality Patient Care Scale (QualPac) used peer evaluators to rate adequacy of care provided in real-life settings (Wandelt & Ager, 1974). The Slater Nursing Competencies Scale also used peer evaluators in actual care settings (Wandelt & Stewart, 1975).

Numerous studies of outcomes linked to quality of care were also conducted in the 1970s. These included development of scales to measure clients' health knowledge and self-care skills (Carey & Posavec, 1978; Gallant & McLane, 1979; Lewis, Firsich, & Parsell, 1979). Patient satisfaction measures were also of interest (Hinshaw & Atwood, 1982).

Focus Away from Quality of Care Issues

After the 1970s there was a decline in the number of quality of care studies. This was not because health care costs were contained or quality of care noticeably improved. On the contrary, health care costs continued to rise, even more steeply than ever, and dissatisfaction with care increased. Rather the emphasis in the 1980s shifted to other, more direct ways of controlling costs. The use of the DRG classification of patients as the basis of prospective payment systems gained attention. Similarly, in nursing there was a resurgence of interest in classification methods, also called case-mix methods, as well as in other management tools. The entire health care industry became preoccupied with becoming more "business-like." Industrial concepts such as productivity were applied to nursing (Davis, Levine, & Sverha, 1986). In short, the emphasis was on efficiency of the delivery of care. In quality of care measurement, process held center stage.

Total Quality Management

In recent years there has been a resurgence of interest in "quality" in the workplace. Programs under the banner of *Total Quality Management* (TQM) have sprung up in all kinds of organizations including health care institutions. TQM was popularized by the work of W. Edwards Deming with Japanese industrial plants. Since Japanese products, especially automobiles and electronics, have attained high ratings for their excellent quality, the management of Japanese companies were seen as models worthy of emulation.

TQM incorporates ideas from quality control sampling methodology, to which Deming, a statistician, had made some contributions in earlier years (1950) and principles of management originated many years ago by theorists of the human relations school (Mayo, 1933). These principles included participative management, democratic leadership styles, and incentives for excellence.

TQM has reawakened interest in quality assessment, although it has not offered any new ideas about how quality should be measured. It has focused attention on the design of quality assurance programs rather than evaluation of quality.

Guidelines for Clinical Practice

In the immediate future and conceivably well into the next century, attention will not primarily be on efficiency or quality of performance, but on the identification of interventions that are clearly beneficial to recipients of health services. Thus, emphasis will be on outcomes of interventions, evaluation of their efficacy through controlled studies such as clinical trials, and determination of the standards of performance for attaining the best outcomes. This emphasis was reinforced in December 1989 when the federal government's Agency for Health Care Policy and Research was established. The Agency is the leading organization in the Medical Treatment Effectiveness Program (MED-TEP) of the U.S. Department of Health and Human Services (Agency for Health Care Policy and Research [AHCPR], 1992; Clinton & Holo-han, 1992). The mission of the Agency is to enhance the quality, appropriateness, and effectiveness of health care services through research and promotion of improvements in clinical practice and in the organization, financing, and delivery of health services.

The Forum for Quality and Effectiveness in Health Care is a major program of AHCPR, responsible for the development and review of clinical practice guidelines that reflect the best current scientific knowledge and judgment about health care interventions for specific health problems. The process for developing guidelines consists of the following:

- Panels of 9 to 15 members are formed and include providers and members of consumer organizations.
- Goals and scope of the guidelines are defined. The framework for determining how outcomes are influenced by various interventions is created.
- Clinical benefits as well as the negative impact of interventions are assessed from completed research and existing databases. Meta-analysis may be used to evaluate effects. Data are combined with expert judgment to create *appropriateness profiles* that are preliminary versions of practice guidelines.
- Health policy issues, including costs, medical liability, limits on resources, and concerns of consumers, providers, and third party payers are assessed.
- Practice guidelines are drafted. They are extensively peer-reviewed, revised, refined, and submitted for further review by providers and consumers before final documents are released.
- Guidelines are disseminated in various formats, including a lengthy technical version, a shorter version, and a quick reference guide. There is also a version for health care consumers.

By the middle of 1993 six practice guidelines had been released: acute pain management, urinary incontinence, pressure ulcers, depression, sickle-cell anemia, and cataracts. Additional guidelines to be released include low back pain and Alzheimer's and related dementias. In addition, practice guidelines are issued by the National Institutes of Health, the Institute of Medicine of the National Academy of Sciences, and professional associations.

To illustrate AHCPR's guidelines, a selection from urinary incontinence in adults includes the following (Urinary Incontinence Guideline Panel, 1992):

- Intermittent catheterization may be appropriate for the management of acute or chronic urinary retention.
- Indwelling catheters may be needed for short-term treatment and for terminally ill patients, but long-term use (more than 2–4 weeks) can lead to secondary problems.
- Biofeedback, used in conjunction with other behavioral treatment techniques, can be useful in the reduction of symptoms associated with UI.
- Long-term use of absorbent products should occur only after a basic evaluation by a health professional.

As is obvious from this sample, guidelines are framed in a more general level of performance than are the quality criteria in a typical quality-of-care measure. There guidelines are more like general principles than recommended procedures. With these as guiding principles, more specific practice guidelines could spell out the proper way of inserting catheters, procedures for monitoring them, what to do when a problem occurs, and so on. If that is done, the result is a manual or textbook on the proper care of people with incontinence. But it is an authoritative textbook, based on best practice and not only on the clinical judgment of the author. Such a textbook could also serve as the source of standards of optimal practice for quality assessment.

The development of practice guidelines is quite useful to the measurement of quality of care, particularly from the perspective of outcomes, because they address the benefits and harms of interventions. As already noted, the evaluation of quality of care involves a comparison of actual practice to a standard or norm. Quality of care represents the extent of deviation from standards or norms. Practice guidelines can provide useful standards for these comparisons because they link specific interventions to specific end results.

Status of Quality of Care Measurement

From the flurry of activity in the 1970s in measurement of quality of care, focus has shifted to evaluation of the efficacy of health care interventions in clinical trials and determination of practice guidelines. Basically, methodology for measuring quality of care has not significantly advanced in the past 20 years. The choice of different measurement approaches remains essentially the same as when they were first described nearly 30 years ago. These approaches are still conceptualized within the well-worn triad of structure, process, and outcome. Collection of data for quality assessment includes a variety of established methods, such as observation, interviewing, structured instruments that collect self-reported data, and use of secondary data from existing databases.

In nursing, a wide choice of valid and reliable instruments are available to assess structure, process, and outcome, individually or in combination. The four-volume collection of measures of nursing performance and outcome, described in the last chapter, contains a varied collection of instruments (Strickland & Waltz, 1988, 1990; Waltz & Strickland, 1988, 1990).

Limitations in Using Outcomes in Quality Measurement

Although much has been said about the virtues of outcomes in quality assessment because they are pragmatic, focusing as they do on benefits and goal achievement, the measurement of outcomes presents some serious problems. Foremost are the intervening and confounding variables that intrude on the relationship between interventions and end results. In addition, the longer the time frame between intervention and outcome, the less accurate conclusions are likely to be, because these variables will have had more time to affect the end results. Then, too, outcomes may be difficult to define operationally, reducing external validity.

Structure and Process in Quality Measurement

Measurement of structure and process generally presents fewer problems than does measurement of outcome. A major dimension of structure is the organization's resources. These are measured in terms of objective data such as budget, numbers and qualification of staff, and physical layout. Process can also be measured objectively in terms of actual staff performance. Considerable data exist to serve as standards or norms of comparison for structural and process evaluations.

An argument for the use of process measures is that because they are causally related to outcomes, they are therefore good predictors of outcomes. The expectation is that good performance leads to good outcomes; or, retrospectively, that good outcomes resulted from good performance. Although examples can undoubtedly be found in nursing where the relationship between process and outcome is nonexistent or perhaps even inverse, more often than not, a positive relationship will be observed. The challenge is to find that a relationship between process and outcome truly exists and that it is appropriate: that the nursing intervention is performed properly and, as a consequence, leads to good results. A medication may be administered correctly—correct dosage, proper timing—but may not do the patient any good. Conversely, the patient may get well despite the fact that the intervention was not correct or was improperly performed.

Use of process measures for evaluation of quality of care, if they are validly related to outcomes, has several advantages. One is that there is quick feedback; there are no long waits for outcomes to appear. Methodology for assessing process can be simple. It is commonly composed of a set of simply scaled and scored behavioral statements or questions, for example, "Was the medication given on time?" Primary data are frequently used in the assessment of process, but secondary data are also useful if available. Use of existing databases reduces costs as well as the time required to collect data. Finally, practice guidelines help in the development of process measures by providing performance standards; they can enhance the validity of evaluations of the nursing process.

The Future of Quality Assessment in Nursing

Future developments in the measurement of quality in nursing will occur in three areas: assessment methodology, practice guidelines, and quality assurance programs.

Assessment Methodology

It is difficult to conceive of any major methodological breakthroughs in quality assessment occurring in the immediate future. The structure-process-outcome triad should continue to provide the accepted framework for categorizing methodology. The variety of approaches to evaluating quality of care from the perspective of process has been fairly well explored. However, outcomes will continue to receive considerable attention, especially in clinical trials and other types of evaluation studies. There is need for development of new outcome measures relevant to nursing, particularly those linked to process. There is also considerable room for the accumulation of pertinent data in accessible databases for use in analytical studies of nursing quality. Finally, there is need for studies that provide in-depth description of the composition of quality of care. Here is where qualitative methodology can play a useful role.

Clinical Practice Guidelines

Defined broadly, a guideline describes the process of health care delivery that will facilitate improvement of health status for those with acute health problems, or slow the decline of health status for those with chronic problems. Guidelines focus on recipients of health services and describe the process by which a desired result is attained. They thus relate process to outcomes. Guidelines help health care providers achieve optimal outcomes by using the best available scientific evidence and professional expertise in the decision making process.

Practice guidelines are also pragmatic; they link quality-assurance and cost-effectiveness to health care management. This will be especially important in the future as solutions to rising health care costs are vigorously pursued and *managed care* becomes more prominent in the future health care system.

Guidelines convert science-based knowledge into clinical action in a form accessible to health care providers. They do not replace professional judgment. On the contrary, they enable professional judgment to inform the provider of the preferred course of action by clarifying health care choices and their consequences for consumers.

Development of practice guidelines for nursing will provide future nurse researchers with a large and challenging agenda of methodological work to be done, as follows:

- A centralized database of existing nursing guidelines should be created that includes normative data as well as data on care standards.
- Nursing variables common to many clinical variables should be consolidated and transformed into practice guidelines.
- A mechanism is needed for capturing clinical knowledge to develop nursing guidelines in areas in which a substantial amount of research has been done. These areas include incontinence, hip

fractures, decubitus ulcers, strokes, rehabilitation, and cardiac recovery.

- The process of developing nursing guidelines should involve expert nurse clinicians, nurse researchers, other health care professionals, and consumers of health care.

The content of research needed to develop comprehensive nursing guidelines is extensive. The future research agenda should give high priority to the following studies:

- Health problems characterized as high-risk, whose solution could have significant benefits for a large number of consumers of health care;
- Problems for which wide variations exist among different treatment options and interventions;
- Problems for which current interventions are costly; and
- Problems for which reliable and valid databases already exist.

Finally, and most importantly, the future research agenda for development of guidelines to improve measurement of quality of nursing must include interventions to promote health and prevent disease. This area is a challenging one. Evaluation of wellness-oriented interventions through outcomes is difficult considering the large amount of time elapsed between input and outcome. There is much room for creativity. The *Year 2000* health objectives can be most helpful in providing outcome measures (U. S. Department of Health and Human Services, 1990, 1991). These objectives must be translated to nursing to enrich future nursing research.

Quality Assurance Programs

Measurement of the quality of care is not an academic exercise. The data have important uses in programs of quality assurance in monitoring ongoing performance, similar to the quality inspection procedures used in manufacturing plants since they were first introduced by Shewhart in 1931. Data on quality of care are also used in the planning of changes in the delivery of care to promote more effective and efficacious services.

Monitoring systems for assuring quality of care generally follow the model defined by the Joint Commission on Accreditation of Healthcare Organizations (Cassidy & Friesen, 1990). Implementation of this model includes the following 10-step process (Joint Commission on Accreditation of Healthcare Organization [JCAHO], 1988, 1990):

anaging the program;

- Assign responsibilities for managing the program;
- Delineate the scope of services provided;
- Specify the most important services;
- Identify indicators and criteria for monitoring the important services;
- Set levels (thresholds) for the indicators which, if exceeded, would initiate an evaluation;
- Collect data for the indicators;
- Evaluate services when thresholds are reached, to pinpoint problems and uncover solutions;
- Initiate actions to correct problems;
- Evaluate the impact of actions in improving services; and
- Disseminate information.

Nurses play key roles in quality assurance programs (Hover & Zimmer, 1978). In many health care organizations, nurses are managers or coordinators of the quality assurance program. Nurses are frequently in collaborative relationships with other health care professionals, especially physicians, in these programs (Hoesing & Kirk, 1990). It can be expected that in the future, nurses will assume an even greater role in the quality assurance process than they have now. This will give methodology for measuring the quality of care from all perspectives—structure, process, and outcome—a high priority in the future research agenda for nursing (Nielsen, 1992).

Chapter 9

Meta-Analysis

Overview

Meta-analysis is neither a research design, like a clinical trial, nor a research approach, like qualitative research. It is a methodology for integrating and evaluating the results of completed research studies through statistical techniques. Although meta-analysis is a relatively new methodology—less than 20 years old—the integration of research results through a literature review has been an important part of research for a very long time. But research reviews are typically *narrative* syntheses of study findings, i.e., "in six studies of the effect of nursing interventions on patients' knowledge of their illness it was found that knowledge increased, etc., etc."

Meta-analysis takes an important step beyond narrative integration. It applies statistical analysis to the combined data of quantitative studies to determine their statistical significance. In meta-analyses of clinical trials, differences in values of outcome measures between treatment and control groups are combined into a pooled *effect size;* e.g., "The results of 20 studies showed that there was a 40% reduction in myocardial infarction in the group taking daily doses of vitamin E." The objective of a meta-analysis is statistical generalization of the combined data.

Meta-analysis is a cost-efficient way of conducting research. Using secondary data from similar studies it increases the strength of study findings in the same way that a larger sample increases *power*. Meta-analysis is especially useful when there is a large pool of replicated studies, as will likely be the case in nursing research in the future. Therefore, it is important to understand what meta-analysis is and how it is used.

What is a Literature Review?

Literature reviews, essential components of the research process, contain narrative discussions of the major methodological and substantive features and conclusions of prior research.

Reviews serve the following useful purposes in research proposals and final reports:

- Provide a meaningful context for the aims and significance of the proposed study by placing it within the context of previous research;
- Help assess the feasibility of the proposed study by revealing possible difficulties;
- Support the undertaking of the proposed study by revealing knowledge gaps, ambiguous areas of information, and questions to be answered;
- Offer guidance on how to operationally define measures to be employed;
- Reveal which methodologies have proved workable and useful and which have not;
- Help formulate the conceptual and theoretical framework;
- Provide a linkage that contributes to the accumulation of knowledge needed for theory development; and
- Provide comparison data for a proposed study and serving as an historical control group.

The procedure for doing a literature review is not standardized. Researchers follow their own preferred style. Reviews are usually terse, highly summarized, and not particularly analytical or evaluative, as demonstrated by the following excerpt from a study of the impact on health personnel supply and education of expanding health promotion programs (Levine, 1982, p. 8):

A thorough search was made of the major reference systems (MED-LINE, ERIC, NHPIC) for literature on the health personnel implications of health promotion and disease prevention programs. Although the literature in the field of prevention is quite extensive, and much of it is of recent origin, linking prevention to personnel requirements, education, utilization, or financing, produced fewer than 100 references mostly oriented to a single discipline, e.g., dentistry and physician extenders. One of the few quantitative assessments was contained in an article by Yoder in the background papers for *Healthy People* which discussed the implications of an increased emphasis on prevention on requirements for health personnel. She concluded that increases in preventive health services would require greater use of non-physician health professionals, particularly nurses.

A literature review is generally free-wheeling, presents little or no synthesized quantitative data, and gives no information on the completeness of coverage or the quality of the material reviewed (Light & Pillemer, 1984). Other criticisms of conventional literature reviews include selective use of data, misleading representations of studies, and no attempt or an incorrect attempt to integrate findings and conclusions into valid generalizations (Jackson, 1978). In short, "chronologically arranged verbal descriptions of research failed to portray the accumulated knowledge," and to rectify this shortcoming it was proposed that "contemporary research reviewing should be more technical and statistical than it is narrative" (Glass, McGaw & Smith, 1981, p. 12).

What is Meta-Analysis?

In its most general definition, meta-analysis means the review and integration of research findings (Glass, McGaw, & Smith, 1981). The prefix "meta" denotes a higher level or more comprehensive analysis. Since the purpose of meta-analysis is to statistically assess the combined results of multiple studies, this methodology is particularly useful in synthesizing clinical trials, and, in fact, this appears to be its most common application. Meta-analysis synthesizes quantitative data from different studies, treating them as replications, thus enlarging the power of the results and permitting more confident generalizations than a single study allows (Glass, 1976).

Meta-analysis is, basically, a method for statistically reanalyzing data from other studies. A good example of the benefits of reanalysis is the research undertaken at the Hawthorne plant of the Western Electric Company in Chicago between 1927 and 1932 (Mayo, 1933). When later reanalyzed, the results led to the discovery of the *Hawthorne Effect* (Roethlisberger & Dickson, 1939).

A new look at data collected by others can uncover fresh insights by using improved statistical techniques. Also, reliability and validity of the findings can be checked. But a reanalysis of a single study is not a meta-analysis. A meta-analysis *combines* quantitative data from multiple studies and applies analytical techniques to test their *significance* and make *statistical generalizations*.

How Has Meta-Analysis Evolved?

Although the term meta-analysis first appeared in the literature in the 1970s, its conceptual foundation was laid many years earlier in the pioneering work of the statisticians Pearson, Fisher, Tippett, Cochran, and others. In 1904 Karl Pearson pooled data from different studies on the relationship between rates of infection from typhoid fever and inoculation and computed an average correlation value. In early editions of their textbooks on statistical methods, Fisher and Tippett described techniques for combining results from several small samples by averaging *probabilities* of obtaining effects rather than computing an average effect size, as in meta-analysis (Fisher, 1925; Tippett, 1931).

In an influential paper Cochran (1937) discussed the limits of combining effects data from different studies and in essence laid the groundwork for the statistical basis of meta-analysis. Mantel and Haenszel (1959) further developed methodology for analyzing data from different studies, extending the work of researchers who were beginning to combine data from independently conducted clinical trials using simple statistical techniques (Dickersin, Higgins, & Meinert, 1990).

The integration of data from disparate sources has a long history in fields such as economics research. Economists studying causes of the business cycle synthesized data from a variety of sources to construct their models. Economic indicators such as the gross national product (GNP) and consumer price index (CPI), computed from data from many different sources, are currently used to analyze a nation's economy. Many researchers in economics and other areas have based entire studies on secondary sources. Computer-aided databases have grown to such an extent that when combined with meta-analysis, they offer a cost-effective way of acquiring new knowledge from secondary sources.

Since the first use of the term in an article by Glass (1976), applications of meta-analysis have grown by leaps and bounds. A number of books on the subject have been published recently including one in nursing (Smith, 1988). Growth has been stimulated by increasing availability of data from completed research studies such as clinical trials (Cooper & Hedges, 1994).

Sources of Data for Meta-Analysis

Before a meta-analysis can be done, the existence of appropriate studies must be determined. The search follows the same procedure as an ordinary literature review. A good starting place is a search of journals and particularly specialty journals. A computerized search using the National Library of Medicine's *Grateful Med*, which any computer with a modem can use, is a cost-effective way of searching journal references.

The question of how many studies are necessary to do a meta-analysis is similar to the question of how large a study sample should be. The obvious answer is: the larger the sample, the greater the confidence in the results, and the more widely the findings can be generalized. A meta-analysis can be done on as few as two studies. The power of two good studies is clearly greater than the power of one. A meta-analysis on a topic of great interest could include many studies. A meta-analysis of treatments for myocardial infarction was based on 182 RCTs, 43 review articles, and 100 textbook chapters (Antman, Lau, Kupelnick, Mosteller, & Chalmers, 1992). This study, incidentally, was conducted in a sequential fashion by progressively adding new data and determining if the additional information altered the conclusions, a procedure similar to sequential sampling.

Used extensively to combine results from RCTs, meta-analysis can also be used to pool data from quasi-experimental studies, including those without a control group. Meta-analysis can even be applied to purely descriptive studies. For example, if there is interest in finding out the nursing dependency levels of older patients newly discharged from acute care hospitals, it might be possible to retrieve data from different studies for a meta-analysis in which average dependency status is the "effect size." It is even possible to conceive of qualitative studies that could be "meta-analyzed."

How is Meta-Analysis Conducted?

The steps in conducting a meta-analysis are similar to the process for conducting any research project (Hunter & Schmidt, 1990). A useful model of the process is *survey research*, in which the objective is to estimate certain parameters of a target population. The population is defined and a sample is selected; data are obtained from each sample member and combined; and estimates of the population parameters are projected from these data using techniques of statistical inference. Similarly, in a meta-analysis, a population is defined; studies are selected that fit the definition; data are extracted, integrated, and summarized; and extrapolations are made to a target population using statistical methodology.

More specifically, the steps in carrying out a meta-analysis are as follows:

1) Determine the General Topical Area for the Analysis

Spell out the domain of the analysis, for example, nursing in critical care units, prevention of bedsores, behavior modification for improving unhealthy lifestyles, and so on. Delineate the variables to be analyzed.

2) Formulate the Theoretical Framework

Describe the theoretical background for the phenomena to be analyzed, if any. Specify the relationships among the variables to be analyzed. Identify any applicable models. Show any linkages to previous research.

3) Specify the Research Questions and/or Hypotheses

Focus on the specific question(s) to be analyzed. For example, the analysis could be directed to the examination of a specific intervention for the prevention of bedsores, the impact of nursing on the reduction of weight among obese persons, or the relationship between RN staffing and mortality rates in critical care units. In descriptive studies the research question could be: What is the prevalence of obesity among RNs? Specifying questions is important because it directs the search that will be made of pertinent studies for the analysis. Vague questions could yield irrelevant data; too narrowly focused questions or hypotheses could limit the usefulness of the analysis.

4) Determine Methodology for Data Retrieval, Data Quality Assessment, and Statistical Tests of Significance

Determine how the search for data bearing on the research questions will be pursued. Identify the computerized databases available for online searches. Describe how the journal article or complete report containing the needed data will be retrieved. Determine criteria for acceptance of data, including the means by which the quality of the data will be evaluated, and design a scoring system for this evaluation. Specify key words for the search, derived from the research questions and hypotheses. Explain the statistical methods, including confidence levels to be used to test for significance. Restate the research questions as statistical hypotheses, if appropriate. Design a data entry form and computer screen for abstracting the data from retrieved documents, including a system for coding the datasets. Determine computer software requirements for performing the statistical tests.

5) Conduct Search for Studies

Using the key words delineated for the research questions, conduct the computerized search for relevant studies. A good place to start is the MEDLINE database of the National Library of Medicine, but other strategies for locating studies will likely have to be pursued (Kirpalani, Schmidt, McKibbon, Haynes, & Sinclair, 1989). Many comprehensive reports of studies remain unpublished, requiring that the researchers be contacted directly to obtain detailed data and other information.

6) Abstract Relevant Data

Assess data for relevance and reliability. Enter data that meet acceptance standards in the data collection form. Determine if data are in a sufficiently consistent and comparable scale to allow application of statistical techniques. If necessary, transform data into a common metric. Enter data into the computer.

7) Perform Statistical Analyses

In a meta-analysis of data from RCTs and other evaluative studies, the analysis focuses on determination of the statistical significance of *effect size* for the combined data (Hedges & Olkin, 1985). Effect size is the average magnitude of differences in outcomes between treatment and control groups in the assembled RCTs. Effect size measures the impact of the intervention; was it efficacious or not? Determining significance of effect size for combined studies is analogous to determining the significance of the difference between arithmetic means, or proportions, or other statistics in a single study. Statistical procedures for pooled data, both parametric and nonparametric, are similar to conventional techniques of statistical significance, requiring only refinements for combining measures from different sized samples and having different variances. The availability of multiple measures also expands the range of techniques that can be applied, including multivariate analysis of variance based on repeated measures.

8) Disseminate Results of the Analysis

Determine the knowledge added by the meta-analysis that is not revealed in individual studies. Indicate the internal and external validity of the data and any limitations of the analysis. Describe the results within a framework of theory, if applicable. Define the boundaries of generalizations of the data. Provide suggestions for applications of results of the analysis and for any further analyses as well as any original research that should be undertaken.

Two Illustrations of the Use of Meta-Analysis

Meta-analysis can be best understood by examining applications of the methodology. Two applications are interesting because they deal with topics of broad public interest. One examines the relationship between chlorination of drinking water and cancer (Morris, Audet, Angelillo, Chalmers, & Mosteller, 1992), the other, the relationship between consumption of oat products and lipid lowering (Ripsin et al.,

1992). They are interesting, too, because the studies which they synthesized used different methodologies. The chlorine study combined data from epidemiological investigations—nonexperimental retrospective studies. The oat bran study combined data from randomized clinical trials. This diversity illustrates the versatility of meta-analysis.

Chlorination and Cancer

Background

Since the turn of the century chlorination has been widely used in the United States in the water purification process, resulting in reduction of water borne diseases such as typhoid fever and hepatitis. About 75% of the nation's water supply is now chlorinated.

In the 1970s concern began to be expressed about the possibility that chlorine, when combined with other organic compounds present in water, was carcinogenic. The focus was particularly on chloroform, the most common byproduct of chlorination, which caused considerable anxiety among the public and led to increased used of bottled water and other substitutes.

A large number of studies were launched to evaluate the chlorination problem using the epidemiological approach of retrospective nonexperimental design based on historical data. The "treatment" group consisted of cases diagnosed with specific forms of cancer. The "control" group consisted mostly of people *without* cancer drawn from the general population. Attempts were made to match cancer cases (the "treatment" group) and controls by important covariates such as age, sex, marital status, and smoking behavior.

The "intervention" studied, through surveys, interviews, and case histories, was exposure to chlorinated water. Exposure meant consumption of chlorinated water or surface (nonwell) water. Nonexposure meant drinking of nonchlorinated water, groundwater, or water treated with both chlorine and ammonia, which prevents introduction of free chlorine into water. Outcome measures were occurrences of morbidity and mortality from cancer. The analysis assessed the statistical significance of any differences in cancer morbidity and mortality between people with and without exposure to chlorinated water.

Research Questions

Was there a relationship between exposure to chlorinated water and neoplastic disease? Did the disease occur in specific sites? If so, which specific sites were most sensitive to exposure? Was the response to chlorinated water associated with amounts of water consumed?

Data Retrieval

MEDLINE was used to search for appropriate studies published from 1966 to 1991. Criteria for inclusion in the search included focus on individual cases, not on aggregated groups, and presence of data on exposure to chlorinated water, morbidity or mortality, and possible confounding variables. Twelve studies were retrieved that concerned the relationship between consumption of chlorinated water and neoplasms, of which two were eliminated because of data inadequacies.

Data Quality Assessment

A key feature of meta-analysis is a rating of the quality of retrieved studies, which is later taken into account in the analysis as a kind of weighting of the importance or strength of the study's findings. A low rating leads to elimination from the analysis. Among the scoring criteria in the chlorination study that characterized high quality were random selection of cases and controls, identification of water source for subjects, adjustment or matching for confounders such as age and sex, and specification of the statistical tests. To promote objectivity of the quality ratings two independent raters evaluated the studies without knowing the journal, authors, institution, or findings. Quality scores for the 10 studies ranged from 43 to 78 within a possible range of 0 to 100. The studies were, thus, of average or somewhat above average quality.

Statistical Test

Meta-analysis was performed on an effect measure known as *relative risk*. A relative risk of 1.00 denotes no difference between the treatment and control groups, that is, no relationship between intervention and outcome. A relative risk significantly greater than 1.00 does show a relationship between intervention and outcome. In the chlorination study, a relative risk exceeding 1.00 meant that cancer *was* associated with intake of chlorinated water. The meta-analysis computed the statistical significance of the relative risk for the 10 studies combined according to site of neoplasm, and also determined the power of these data.

Analysis and Interpretation of Findings

The relative risk for two sites was significantly greater than 1.00: bladder and rectum. Moreover, there was a relationship between the amount of exposure and incidence of neoplasm. Controlling possible confounding variables such as smoking and occupation did not affect the relationship. Clinical validity was supported by the finding that colon and other cancers were not associated with chlorinated water intake. The bladder and rectum store the body's waste products; the colon does not. Storage lengthens the period of exposure of these organs to potential ill effects of chloroform.

Value of the Meta-analysis

The meta-analysis produced considerably more revealing information than the inconclusive results of the 10 individual studies; only three found a statistically significant relative risk for bladder cancer and only two for rectal cancer. Projecting relative risk to the United States population as a whole yielded the following substantively significant conclusion: An incidence each year of 4,200 cases of bladder cancer and 6,500 cases of rectal cancer due to the drinking of chlorinated water.

Limitations of the Meta-analysis

A meta-analysis is only as good as the studies on which it is based. The chlorination studies, as examples of epidemiological research, were adequate, but they were not RCTs. How could the RCT method have been used to answer the questions posed in these studies? RCTs have limited use in investigating environmental and other problems; the research conditions are impossible to simulate in an RCT, confounding factors are difficult to control, and many years can elapse between exposure and response. RCTs of the impact of health promotion and disease prevention programs on health status would be especially difficult to do, not only because of the extensive lag between intervention and outcome, but because of the large sample needed to detect significance (Thornquist, Patrick, & Omenn, 1991).

In a meta-analysis of nonexperimental studies, the question becomes one of external validity. How extensively can the findings be extrapolated? In the absence of true causal research, generalizations should be tempered with caveats; the results, although promising, are suggestive and not definitive. In the case of the chlorination meta-analysis, although findings were not conclusive, they raised the possibility of a link between water quality and health status. The appropriate conclusion could well be that chlorination, proven effective in eliminating water borne diseases, should be modified with ammonia to eliminate chlorine's bad effects.

Oat Products and Lipid Lowering

Background

In the 1960s, evidence began to accumulate from several uncontrolled studies that addition of oat bran to the diet lowered total blood cholesterol in human subjects. Because high cholesterol levels had already been implicated as a risk factor in the development of heart disease, by far the leading cause of death in the United States, a number of clinical trials were conducted to study the relationship between oat bran and cholesterol.

These trials were quite straightforward. A treatment group was fed a special diet that included a specific amount of oat bran or oatmeal; the control group's diet did not. Some trials had multiple treatment groups, including a test of the effects of wheat as well as oat bran. The trials were unblinded and it would be hard to conceive how the intervention could have been disguised. The outcome measure was total blood cholesterol level. Results were quite variable; some studies found significant declines in cholesterol levels in members of the treatment group, whereas others did not. The purpose of the meta-analysis was to integrate the results of individual RCTs to assess the combined effect size.

Because RCTs are conducted under quite strict procedures, they lend themselves very nicely to a meta-analysis. Results of individual trials were not consistent, however, due to study variations. Some trials used oatmeal; others used oat bran. The trials also varied by age and gender of study subjects, as well as the length of time that the oat product was administered, from less than a month to 12 weeks. Moreover, the daily quantity of oat product ingested differed, and the baseline blood cholesterol levels of subjects varied. Finally, there is the effect of the lack of blinding.

In assembling disparate and contradictory data such as these, considerable attention has to be paid to making them as comparable as possible by identifying confounding variables. This study demonstrated a good feature of meta-analysis; that is, it provides a systematic approach to comparing and assessing results of studies with different design characteristics.

Research Hypotheses

The meta-analysis examined a number of hypotheses. One addressed the lipid-lowering effect of oat products, and held that the effect is increased with greater consumption of oat products (dose/response relationship). Another was that persons with higher initial total cholesterol levels and older women would show greater reductions from the oat bran than others.

Data Retrieval

In conducting a meta-analysis of studies such as these, in which many confounding and intervening variables can influence results, the original studies have to be reanalyzed, so it is important to obtain as much detail as possible. The literature search in this study consisted of two main approaches. First, oat product trials published as of March 1991 were retrieved from MEDLINE. Second, a list of unpublished trials was compiled and the principal investigators contacted for possible inclusion of their data. All investigators were asked to supply additional raw data that could be used in the analysis.

Twenty trials were identified by the search process, of which 12 had been published. One unpublished trial provided no information; therefore, 19 trials were available to analyze.

Data Quality Assessment

In order to be entered into the meta-analysis the data had to meet certain criteria. These included, in addition to a proper RCT design, the clear identification and separation of treatment groups that tested other interventions, such as wheat bran or special low-fat, low-cholesterol diets. Also, the data for the calculation of the combined effect size had to be adequate. Ten trials met the quality criteria, and because some had multiple treatment groups, 19 individual effect sizes were included.

Statistical Test

The data were subjected to numerous statistical adjustments and analyses. The objective was to use the pooled data to test the statistical significance of differences in total cholesterol level (effect size) between subjects who ate oat products and controls who did not. A statistic known as *Keys scores* was used in the analysis to measure the effect of dietary changes, that is, the substitution of carbohydrates for dietary fats and cholesterol.

Analysis and Interpretation of Findings

The researchers carefully interpreted the findings, concluding that there was strong support for a relationship between consumption of oat products and total blood cholesterol. Specifically, the meta-analysis showed that 3 grams per day of soluble fiber from oat bran or oatmeal reduced total cholesterol level 5 to 6 mg/dl, a rather modest effect. However, a greater reduction in the total cholesterol level occurred from ingesting oat bran for those who had high cholesterol levels initially.

Extrapolating the results of the meta-analysis to the total United States population, it was estimated that a 1% reduction in the cholesterol level could lower the death rate from heart disease by 2%. In that context, even a small reduction in total blood cholesterol level would have a significant impact on the health status of large numbers of people. However, generalizations such as these must be stated with appropriate caveats. How can external validity be established? The subjects in the 10 studies analyzed were not a random sample drawn from a specified target population. Therefore, the investigators recommended that a large-scale clinical trial lasting at least 6 months be conducted to verify the results of this meta-analysis which, in essence, served as an exploratory study.

Comments on the Meta-analysis

The write-up of the meta-analysis contains a fairly lengthy discussion of limitations. The investigators discuss what is called *file drawer* bias, which results when pooled estimates are based solely on published reports that are not representative of the universe of studies. Also, the design of individual studies were varied in duration of the trials, selection of study subjects, and procedures for drawing blood. Furthermore, there was lack of blinding, which the investigators did not discuss.

Strengths and Limitations of Meta-Analysis

As these two studies have clearly shown, meta-analysis is a useful method for the integration and analysis of studies of similar phenomena. Although its most useful application appears to be in the synthesis of quantitative data from empirical studies, many aspects of the meta-analysis process can be used to integrate qualitative data. By providing a systematic approach to reviewing research literature in general, it can help improve the collection and analysis of data, especially if it is done within a theoretical framework that helps to focus on the relevancy of the data.

The concept of quasi-clinical trials was mentioned to denote possible modifications of RCTs to make them more applicable to nursing research. A modified meta-analysis is also conceivable that could be more useful to nursing research than the traditional method. These modifications are discussed in the next chapter.

Critics warn that the results of all meta-analyses have to be interpreted very cautiously (Thompson & Pocock, 1991). As is true for any other research methodology, meta-analysis has both strengths and limitations that can be summarized as follows:

Strengths

- Using data from other studies, meta-analysis is cost- effective. Answers to research questions can be obtained in a fraction of the time and with considerably less expense than carrying out an original study. Conceivably, much of the work in carrying out a meta-analysis can be done by one person with a computer and appropriate literature search and statistical analysis software.
- It increases the power of the primary studies by enlarging the sample. In so doing, it can identify statistically significant results that individual studies with lesser power cannot.
- Enlarging the sample can provide wider scope for the generalization of findings. Thus, if one primary study had only men in its sample, another included only women, and a third study included both men and women and also had a wider geographic scope, the target population can be significantly expanded beyond that of a single study by combining the data from the three studies.
- Meta-analysis produces a more intensive and critical analysis of a study than does a regular literature review. The process calls for a

systematic evaluation of the quality of the study's methodology and data. Restricting the analysis to high-quality studies enhances both the internal and external validity of the findings.

- A meta-analysis reanalyzes the data of the primary study and new findings can emerge. Or, a study can be redesigned on an *ex post facto* basis, such as analyzing selected parts of the individual studies, to provide a fresh perspective on the results. For example, a meta-analysis could be done on the effectiveness of all RN staffs. Only those studies in which minimum preparation of the staffs was a baccalaureate degree could be included in the analysis; the analysis could include only mixed staffs; or mixed staffs could be compared to all-degree RNs. In any case, the meta-analysis provides a way of answering research questions that the primary studies did not.

- A meta-analysis provides guidance in the planning of further research. It can stimulate ideas about new questions and hypotheses by revealing gaps in research. Insights gained by the critical analysis of the quality of the completed studies help to improve the methodological approach to be used in additional studies.

- Meta-analysis increases the usefulness of a study. A lot of hard work must go into the conduct of research. Moreover, good research data in nursing are quite scarce. A technique that takes these hard-earned data and uses them for additional investigations has much to recommend it. This becomes especially important as money for research becomes less available.

Limitations

- A meta-analysis is only as good as the quality of studies it includes (Brown, 1991). A meta-analysis can obtain new insights not revealed by the original studies, but if the studies are weak, validity will suffer.

- Reports of studies are sometimes deficient in information necessary to carry out a meta-analysis adequately. A study may be good, but a poor write-up will diminish its usefulness in a meta-analysis.

- A meta-analysis looks backwards because it uses completed studies as its "primary" data. Some of the studies may have been conducted a number of years ago. In this fast-changing world, old data may not be relevant to present day problems, let alone future ones. Moreover, because many important current problems have not previously been researched, there are no data that could be assembled for a meta-analysis. Only a new study will supply the needed information.

- Many studies appropriate for a meta-analysis are narrowly focused. Also, studies may use effect measures that are not very meaningful. Thus, although the meta-analyses of these studies may find statistically significant effects, they may not have much practical importance.
- There is a literalness to meta-analysis because it is frequently used to investigate causal relationships by dwelling on direct evidence; for example, whether all RN staffs provide better quality nursing care than do mixed staffs. However, in order to produce useful findings, many research problems may need a more subtle approach including use of projective techniques.
- Several technical difficulties affect the validity of a meta-analysis. First, the ratings of the quality of studies are subjective. This can let a poor study slip through that reduces the accuracy of the effect size. Second, validity of the effect size is diminished when it is calculated from studies with different sampling errors and different methodologies, including diverse scales of measurement. Third, control of confounding variables in the meta-analysis depends on how well that was accomplished in the primary studies. Sometimes it is not possible to tell how the investigators addressed the problem of confounding and intervening variables from the write-up of the study.
- Although meta-analysis is reputed to be applicable to all kinds of studies, statistical and nonstatistical, the major use appears to be in synthesizing epidemiological studies and clinical trials, which are examples of quantitative research (Cordray, 1990; Mosteller, 1990). There is no agreement as to whether quantitative analysis is its only use. Considering that the "analysis" in meta- analysis is statistical analysis, it would seem that its main use is indeed in quantitative research (Hedges & Olkin, 1985).

The Future of Meta-Analysis in Nursing Research

Meta-analysis has become a buzz-word in the research world. It has even developed some characteristics of a cult. It has been used where an ordinary literature review could have served just as well, if not better. And it has been used where it was totally inappropriate.

Despite its limitations, meta-analysis is a good technique with a useful role to play in research. *However, it should not be made to do more than its capabilities.* The question is, how useful can it be to nursing research? The answer depends on where nursing research is going in the future, because up to this time it seems that a full-blown meta-analysis, culminating in statistical analyses of effect sizes, has limited applicability. This is so because there have not been very many studies of "effects" in nursing, the data from which could be pooled for a meta-analysis. An example of a meta-analysis conducted by nurse researchers underscores this point (Goode et al., 1991).

In contrast to medical research in which many different interventions have been evaluated in large numbers of repeated clinical trials, nursing research is still in many ways, in its early stages of development and decidedly less homogeneous. Consider the fact that in fiscal year 1993 the federal government's National Center for Nursing Research (now the National Institute of Nursing Research), the major funding source for nursing research, supported approximately 240 projects that varied greatly in subject matter and methodological characteristics (National Center for Nursing Research [NCNR], 1992c). In contrast, one meta-analysis found nearly 240 studies of therapies for a single medical problem, myocardial infarction (Antman, Lau, Kupelnick, Mosteller, & Chalmers, 1992).

It seems that meta-analysis would be of greatest value to nursing research in providing a disciplined process for reviewing and synthesizing completed research that does not necessarily have as its main objective a statistical analysis of effect size. In the future more applications of meta-analysis to descriptive studies can be expected (Reynolds, Timmerman, Anderson, & Stevenson, 1992). Easing of the statistical requirements and objectives of meta-analysis would make it possible to include fewer and more heterogeneous studies in the analysis and to redirect the study selection standards away from purely statistical criteria such as control of variables, randomization of study subjects, and specification of tests to more qualitative criteria. The end result of the analysis could then be a synthesis of the knowledge gained from the studies, expressed qualitatively as well as quantitatively.

In the future, as evaluation research in nursing continues to expand into clinical areas, and as studies that are comparable in aims, subject matter, and methodology become more prevalent, opportunities to apply the formal meta-analysis technique will surely increase. In the meantime, a review of the nursing research literature should incorporate those features of meta-analysis that help to increase the validity and usefulness of the synthesized information.

Chapter 10

Improving Nursing Research Methods

The Role of Methodologies in Research

"Research methodology" refers to the methods for collecting, processing, and analyzing research data. Methodologies in nursing research have steadily evolved over the past 40 years from rather simple approaches to collecting and analyzing data to use of sophisticated methods and designs. Methodology is a dominant theme in the nursing research literature. Many studies are more notable for what they say about methodology than for their substantive findings.

What does an assessment of this prolific use of methodology reveal? Has methodology become the tail wagging the dog? Have nurse researchers become too enamored of methodology? Has too much effort been put on methodology to the detriment of advancement of the substance and content of nursing science? Is a better balance between methodology and content needed? It is time to examine what methodology has worked best and which will serve the needs of future nursing research.

Variety of Topics

Methodology has been so varied in nursing research because the content of studies has been so diverse. To assess what is happening in the nursing research world, over 100 articles reported in the major nursing research and scholarly journals during 1992 were reviewed.

The first impression from the review was that recent nursing studies have included a dazzling array of subject matter. The topics, sampled from eight journals, *Nursing Research*, *Western Journal of Nursing Research*, *Research in Nursing and Health*, *Applied Nursing Research*, *Image*, *Journal of Advanced Nursing*, *Advances in Nursing Science*, and *Nursing Science Quarterly*, include the following:

- Low-vision adults;
- Skin problems;
- Long-term psychiatric patients;
- Coping behavior;
- Locus of control;
- AIDS;
- Circadian rhythms;
- Infertility;
- Urine stream;
- Obese children;
- Loneliness; and
- Breast self-examination.

Coincidentally, the grants supported by the National Center for Nursing Research (NCNR, now NINR), now nine as of October 1992, include a similar diversity of topics, as the following small sample shows:

- Weight management;
- AIDS;
- Hip surgery;
- Myocardial infarction;
- Pressure sores;
- Battered women;
- Incontinence;
- Adolescent parents;
- Alzheimer's disease;
- Pain in children;

- Renal transplant outcomes; and
- Cystic fibrosis.

The variety of topics pursued by nurse researchers has had several consequences. First, data in many subject matter areas tend to be extensive, and not intensive. The lack of replicated studies has impeded the development of knowledge bases. Second, because the studies are so varied, it is difficult to see what the priorities in research are. This situation raises many questions. Why does the research agenda seem to be heading in all directions? What is important? What are the knowledge needs to develop a nursing science? Who decides the direction of nursing research? Where does the guidance for a coherent research policy originate? Why is nursing research less directed towards "pure" scientific research and more directed towards practical solutions to problems?

Variety of Methodologies

The diversity of study topics pursued in nursing research has had an interesting result. It has led to a variety of applications of research methodologies to nursing topics. Nursing research employs the entire gamut of research designs, from descriptive surveys to highly controlled randomized clinical trials, as well as the less structured approaches of qualitative research. Methods of data collection and analysis are similarly diverse. The sampling of the eight journals revealed not only a wide array of topics, but, also, a textbook-full collection of measuring instruments, scales, and statistical techniques.

Weaknesses in the Use of Research Methodology

The evolution of nursing research shows a trend toward greater complexity in the methodologies used. This would be fine if the studies produced better results—richer data, better designs, more profound answers to questions. However, this has not necessarily been the case. Part of the problem has to do with methodological weaknesses of the studies. But this is not meant to condemn nursing research. From a methodological standpoint, nursing research is at least as good as research in related fields. Sechrest and Hannah (1990), in an assessment of the importance of nonexperimental data in testing causal relationships in health research, reviewed 100 studies published in health services research journals. More than 50% of the studies had deficiencies in sampling, measurement, and external validity. One-third had unjustified conclusions, for the most part meaning that the researchers claimed unwarranted cause-and-effect relationships. The studies in the eight nursing journals revealed similar methodological problems, the most persistent of which included the following:

Measurement Problems

Studies provided minimal information on validity and reliability of the data. Although construct validity was frequently mentioned, the description of the study variables was not sufficient for the reader to make a judgment.

Purposive and Convenience Samples

The majority of studies used purposive, non-randomly selected samples, typically persons receiving services in the institution at the time of the study, such as patients in a hospital unit, mothers attending a prenatal care program, persons in a physical fitness program, or students in a school of nursing. There is no prohibition against using a "convenience" sample as long as the limitation on making statistical generalizations is recognized. A researcher is free to project study findings to a larger population without using statistical inference, but these generalizations are based on judgment, not on the laws of chance.

No Assessment of Power

Even when samples were randomly drawn, power analysis to determine the probability of making type II errors was not reported. However, it seems that too much is made of the concept of power in nursing research. Power tests certainly have a place in randomized clinical trials. This type of research is too costly to be invalidated by inadequate samples. But many nursing studies differ from controlled clinical trials. First, because they do not utilize random sampling, the statistical model underlying the concept of statistical power does not really apply. Moreover, because measurements are frequently based on nominal or ordinal scales, they are quantitatively soft and nonparametric, making the calculation of the power function a questionable exercise.

Uses and Misuses of Statistical Tests of Significance

The basic tools of statistical inference are determining confidence intervals for a sample measure, known as statistical estimation, and conducting tests of significance.

Statistical Estimation

As has been noted, the fundamental purpose of statistical inference is to compute the amount of *sampling* error in measures of variables studied. In descriptive, univariable analysis, confidence intervals are computed for a summary measure of the variables, such as an arithmetic mean of the individual measures. A confidence interval is the range within which the true summary measure value for the whole population lies at a stated level of probability. The probability, or confidence level, very often selected is 95%. This means that 95 times out of 100 the population value will lie within the confidence interval, which is the value of the sample summary measure plus and minus twice the value of its standard error. The standard error is a measure of sampling error determined from a formula in which, basically, the average variability of the values of individual sample measures is divided by the size of the sample.

Statistical Test of Significance

Tests of significance of *differences* in the values of multiple sample summary measures, as in evaluating differences between the mean values of outcome measures for the treatment and control groups in a clinical trial, are actually extensions of the method of computing confidence intervals for a single summary measure. In fact, instead of applying tests of significance, confidence intervals could be computed for the value of each outcome measure. They then could be superimposed to determine the extent of overlap. If the intervals do not or only barely overlap, the conclusion is that the measures probably came from different populations, i.e., they are significantly different (from a statistical perspective). Thus, it is concluded that the treatment had a significant effect at the confidence level selected.

Tests of significance of differences between outcome measures are analogous to comparisons of confidence intervals. The difference between treatment and control group outcomes (effect size) is divided by the standard error of the summary measure. According to the laws of chance the probability that the difference will exceed the standard error by *two* is five times out of 100, or 0.05, the level of significance commonly used. Thus, if the value of the ratio is two or more, the conclusion is that the treatment and control groups represent different populations; in other words, the treatment had a significant effect on the study subjects.

The purpose of this discussion is to stress that statistical tests of significance and confidence intervals are, strictly speaking, *only* applicable to data that have been generated through a random process—random sampling or random allocation—to which the laws of probability apply. In most of the studies reviewed in the eight nursing journals this rule was ignored. Study after study used what can best be labeled "convenience samples," yet the analysis of the data employed tests of significance based on probability models, including very sophisticated ones such as the analysis of variance (ANOVA) and the analysis of covariance (ANCOVA). Moreover, repeated tests were employed while ignoring that the Type I error rate (0.05), the error of finding significance in study data by chance alone, is inflated when many tests are run of the same measure. At the 0.05 level this could happen five times in every 100 tests. Repeated testing of the same measures in an effort to find statistical significance is called "fishing" for significance. Through this approach, sooner or later, significance will be found by chance alone.

Justification of the use of tests of significance when data are not obtained from random samples perhaps rests on the notion that chance (random factors) plays a role in any study. Patients in a hospital, nurses in a home care agency, students in a school of nursing, happen to be there by chance when the study was conducted. They were not deliberately selected as would be, say, a subject in a study of client satisfaction who was chosen because of a known good opinion of the agency.

Although "accidental" selection of study subjects is purported to be like a random sample in that it is an *unbiased* sample, the two methods are not the same. One key difference is that a random sample is selected from a larger *target* population. Statistical extrapolations of data thus can be made from sample to population. *Statistical* generalizations cannot be made from nonrandom samples. Strictly speaking, only generalizations based on the judgment of the researcher are permissible. So why apply tests of significance when they are not needed?

To justify inferences from nonrandom samples, the idea of a *hypothetical* or *conceptual universe* has been advanced. Its premise is that even nonrandomly chosen subjects are drawn from a hypothetical universe and are "representatives" of members of that universe. To repeat, it is the researcher's prerogative to extrapolate data from a nonrandom sample to a defined universe. However, the generalization cannot be supported by statistical inferences, only by the researcher's judgment.

Other Problems in the Use of Statistical Tests

In addition to misuse and overuse of statistical inference, the review of studies in the eight nursing journals revealed still other problems:

Attributing Causality

There is a tendency to interpret statistical significance as proof of causality. If the effect size is statistically significant, it is likely to be attributed to the intervention as the causal agent. But even in the most highly controlled studies, a confounding variable could be the actual causal agent; or a Type I error may be responsible. Statistical significance denotes a *relationship* among variables, but not necessarily a *causal* one.

Statistical Significance is Not an Indicator of How Good a Study Is

The attitude of some researchers is that because they have found statistical significance (or because they ran high-powered tests) therefore their study must be good. It may seem to some that the presence of large amounts of data in a study report preceded by elegant mathematical formulas puts the seal of excellence on the study. That a study with a profusion of statistical data and statistical tests is not necessarily of high quality is not only borne out by a critical perusal of reported studies, but by the work of qualitative researchers, who have produced many fine research reports without a trace of quantitative data.

Wrong Statistical Tests are Used

Even when random sampling is used and the data can properly be subjected to statistical tests, the wrong test may be employed. This occurs in two situations. First, each method of sampling has its own formula for calculating sampling error. A simple unrestricted random sample uses, appropriately, a simple formula. A multistage sample with stratification uses a more complex formula. Often, though, a simple formula is used when a more complex one is called for.

Second, each of the different tests of significance, especially para-metric tests, require that certain assumptions be met by the data. In addition to the requirement of randomness and that the measure-ments be independent of each other, e.g., the temperature of subject A is not affected by subject B's raging fever, other requirements and assumptions may also apply. For example, when ANOVA is used, there is the assumption that the errors are independent random values from *normally* distributed populations. There is also the requirement that the scale of measurement for the outcome measure (dependent variable) be a quantitatively scaled *continuous* one. Other tests have their own requirements and assumptions. However, as these require-ments are often ignored, the wrong test is being used. A way around this is to use nonparametric tests that, although they result in some loss of information, do not violate statistical theory because they re-quire minimal assumptions about the data.

The Level of Statistical Significance Does Not Necessarily Signify the Strength of a Relationship

Even if the difference in outcomes for the treatment and control groups is highly significant, it does not necessarily mean that the ef-fect of the intervention is stronger than if the difference were less sta-tistically significant. Getting significance at the 0.0001 level may well be the result of a good design that minimizes errors. Moreover, differ-ences in outcomes could be small, yet, statistically very significant, well beyond the 0.05 level. This, then, could be a case of statistical significance without practical significance. If a sample is large enough, even small differences become statistically significant be-cause of the high power of the test.

At the risk of sounding repetitive, a test, no matter how highly sig-nificant its results, signifies whether there is a *statistical* relationship, not a *causal* one. The intrusion of extraneous variables haunts every study. Causality is not absolutely proven by the data of a single study, but is confirmed by multiple studies.

Temporality of Statistical Significance

Finding statistical significance in data today does not necessarily mean that the research questions or hypotheses are answered forever. Even highly significant findings are subject to change. Thus, in gen-eralizing results of a study, there should be some constraint on how far into the future they are extrapolated. After all, a study is conducted not only *with* a sample of study subjects, but *at* a sample of time. Data may be collected during only a few weeks of the year. Could this sample of time be representative of all weeks of the year? Of years into the future?

Few of the studies reported in the eight journals addressed the limitation of the "time sample." This is not surprising because study limitations are rarely discussed—not only the temporal issue, but other important issues, such as the implications of using a convenience sample; analytical problems created by nonresponse, dropouts, and other causes of missing data; shortcomings in validity and reliability of data-collecting instruments; and consequences of failures to meet the assumptions of the statistical tests used.

There is another side to the issue of temporality. Sometimes a study is terminated before statistical significance is revealed even though it may really be there. This is fundamentally a Type II error in which the sample was too small, that is, of insufficient power, to detect significance. But the problem may not necessarily be not having a large enough sample. In prospective evaluation studies such as clinical trials, sufficient time might not be allowed for the intervention to exert an impact on the outcome measure. In other words, the time sample was not large enough. Clinical trials of drugs and other therapies are beset with this problem. Cholesterol-lowering drugs, for example, may take a fairly long time to affect LDL or HDL levels in the blood of human subjects. Terminating a trial too early loses valuable information by truncating the data. Extending it, however, not only increases costs of the study but, as in all lengthy longitudinal studies, raises the chances of sample attrition.

Methodological Issues For The Future

The assessment of nursing research reported in recent journals has perhaps dwelled too much on deficiencies. In fairness to nurse researchers, it must be pointed out that they have carved out a difficult area. They are dealing with an array of complex problems for which the *practicable* methodological approaches are mainly nonexperimental or quasi-experimental designs. These designs present many challenges that must be overcome if the studies are to produce valid and reliable results. Although the previous discussion may have given a negative impression, nurse researchers should be complimented for pursuing important research topics in order to strengthen the scientific basis of nursing and improve the quality of care.

How Methodology can be Improved

The remainder of this chapter will shift to a more positive and forward-looking direction. The central question to be addressed is: Considering the current state of the art in the use of methodology in nursing research, what can be done in the future to increase methodological creativity and productivity? Before attempting to answer this question, a necessary preamble is a brief discussion of some of the recommendations for methodological improvements from the Sechrest and Hannah (1990) evaluation that have implications for improving nursing research. The authors compiled an imposing list of recommendations for strengthening research methodology from a survey of reviewers of proposals for health services research grants. These extended to over 40 different aspects of research purpose, design, and methodology. The most pertinent recommendations for improvement of nursing research include the following:

- The literature review should show the connection of the proposed study with previous studies. The significance of the proposed study should be fully described. The research question(s) should be stated with precision.
- A conceptual framework for the study, including models, hypotheses, and research questions should help the selection and design of appropriate methodology.
- If previously explored phenomena are to be studied, a different methodological approach might yield more productive results than simple replication of old methods.
- All variables should be clearly and precisely described. Operational definitions are essential. New measures of variables need not be developed if valid and reliable measures exist. All new instruments must be tested for validity and reliability. Outcome measures should be precise and relevant. Scales should be refined and meaningful.
- Data collectors must be adequately trained. Interrater reliability should be evaluated. Attention must be given to problems associated with recall data.
- The sampling plan should be clearly described. Whenever possible sample selection should be random. Problems of sample attrition, refusals to participate, missing data, and nonresponse should be addressed during the early stages of the research. Es-

timation of desirable sample size should include power calculations, if applicable.

- Problems of using retrospective data should be considered prior to data collection.
- Limitations of the study, particularly those pertaining to collection, analysis, and interpretation of data, should be identified. Conclusions relating to causality should be tempered by the ability of the research methodology to control intervening and confounding variables. The researcher's knowledge and judgment should guide conclusions about the substantive importance of the results.

Methodology for Nursing Research

The principles and techniques of research methodology are not engraved in concrete. There is considerable flexibility in planning and conducting research for modifying existing methods in order to enrich the data collected and their analysis. In actual practice, however, with the exception of instruments to collect data, there appears to be little methodological adventurousness in most areas of research. In medical research, for example, the "in thing" is the randomized clinical trial (RCT), as perusal of medical journals will show.

In the review of the eight nursing journals a preponderance of articles about a favored methodology was not discerned. In fact, the literature was quite eclectic. RCTs appeared in a few articles (or at least CTs) as did just about every kind of research methodology including, of course, qualitative research. The general impression given by many of the articles is of a textbookish approach to research. This has its compensations. We can assume that well-used methodology has been thoroughly tested for validity and reliability. Moreover, replicated methodology can lead to confirmation of previous results and contribute to the accumulation of scientific knowledge.

Thus, there are good arguments not to stray far afield in methodology development and use. Construction of the tools of research is a specialized line of work. Although some research projects are concerned only with design of methodology, they usually receive lower priority scores than do studies of substantive problems. The attitude seems to be: Leave methodology to the methodologists and get on with the pursuit of important research questions.

It is probably true that nurse researchers have left their imprint on research methodology. Researchers have revised, refined, and reinvented methodology that is customized for nursing. Except in the area of instrument development and possibly in qualitative methods, the contributions are hard to see immediately. Only an in-depth analysis will bring this to light. The appearance in recent years of new research journals in nursing, such as *Applied Nursing Research* and *The Journal of Nursing Measurement*, should provide wider dissemination of methodological developments.

It is not proposed here that an all-out effort be mounted to construct customized and highly specialized methodology for nursing research. There is no evidence that this would lead to a significant improvement in the quality and significance of research findings. It could also deflect resources away from important problems. What is suggested is that a low-key effort to improve methodology, one that brings creativity to the task and explores ways of increasing research productivity, will have a good impact on both the quality and quantity of nursing research.

The closing sections of this chapter will present a few suggestions for improving the use of research methodology in nursing. This will serve as a summary of and conclusions about future directions of methodology. The suggestions are guided by the objective of increasing creativity and productivity in the selection and use of research methodology. They are down-to-earth, not difficult, and can be implemented within the normal process of research.

Some suggestions have already been discussed or at least implied in previous chapters of this book. For the most part they are techniques that have been found useful in other fields of research. They may have even been used in some nursing studies. The suggestions will be discussed in three main areas of research methodology: research design, data collection/processing, and data analysis/interpretation. Data analysis refers to the application of statistical and other techniques to the compilation, summarization, and testing of the collected data. "Interpretation" refers to the researcher's understanding of the meaning and importance of the findings and their extrapolation and dissemination to the nursing community and the world at large.

Increasing Productivity and Creativity in Future Nursing Research

Every researcher writing a proposal is concerned about including that "extra something" that will attract the attention of the reviewer. In the extremely competitive world of research, made even more so by the scarcity of resources, it is most important that a proposal stands out. If the methodology described in a proposal is creative and productive, it will be appealing as long as it does not go off in an eccentric and confusing direction.

Simply stated, creativity refers to an imaginative approach that departs from conventional practices, yet achieves better results. Productivity means achievement of better results without increase in resources. Some methodological approaches combine creativity and productivity. It is not the intention of the following review to present an exhaustive list of suggestions, but only to comment on a few major ones to illustrate the potential for methodology enhancement.

Research Design

Quasi-Clinical Trials

As clinical nursing research has expanded there has been increased interest in conducting clinical trials. Fully controlled RCTs are expensive, time-consuming, and narrowly focused. There are a few notable examples of a nursing RCT, but even these have had to deviate from the ideal design, notably in their inability to apply the double-blind technique and in the severe loss of study subjects over the long time period required to obtain outcome measurements.

Much is being written lately about loosening some of the controls found in the classic clinical trial. Although this would possibly sacrifice some precision in data results, costs would be reduced, as well as some of the many pressures alleviated which are generated in the attempt to comply with the strict RCT design. The term *quasi-clinical trial* could be used, not pejoratively, but to distinguish a modified clinical trial from the ideal RCT model, which in any case is not really a practical design for many conceivable nursing studies.

Historical Controls

A simplification of the RCT that has received little attention in nursing research is the use of *historical controls*. Instead of assigning study subjects to a control group, this method uses results of other studies for comparison with the treatment group. This reduces the number of study subjects required by eliminating the control group. Alternatively, the treatment group could be enlarged to increase the power of test results. Of course, secondary data must be comparable, especially in the characteristics of study subjects, nature of interventions, and outcome measures. As nursing databases expand in the future through replication of studies, use of historical controls will become more practicable.

Crossover Designs and Sequential Sampling

There are other ways to conduct clinical trials and other kinds of experimental and quasi-experimental research with fewer study subjects without sacrificing power. The *crossover design*, in which a study subject sequentially serves as a member of both treatment and control groups, is an example. O'Hare (1992) used this design in an evaluation of different models of discharge planning rounds. Another efficient technique is *sequential sampling*, in which the size of the sample is determined by treatment results and not fixed in advance (Armitage, 1975). Techniques such as these, although potentially advantageous, do have limitations that must be fully understood by the researcher before using them.

Large, Simple Trials

Because RCTs are so expensive, recent suggestions have been made for modifications that would relax design aspects that are especially resource-intensive. The concept of large, simple trials resembles meta-analysis in that data are brought together from a number of comparable studies, except that in large, simple trials the data are collected prospectively. In these studies RCT procedures are relaxed and data collection is kept to the minimum necessary to obtain useful information.

Large simple trials provide outcome data in a shorter time frame than can multicenter trials which are simultaneously conducted in a few sites using strict RCT methodology. For example, in 1991 the Heart, Lung and Blood Institute of the National Institutes of Health conducted a trial of the drug digoxin on patients with congestive heart failure in 320 sites in the United States (Brown, 1992). Many of the sites were physicians' offices. Data collection was kept to a bare minimum. Three simple outcome measures were used: episodes of hospitalization, incidence of heart attacks, and death. By enrolling 8,000 subjects there was assurance that a sufficient number of deaths would occur among study subjects in a relatively short period of time, so that if the drug were truly effective, significant differences in deaths between treatment and control subjects could be detected. The conventional clinical trial, using smaller samples, would have had to extend the period of data collection over a longer and more costly time span.

In essence, large, simple clinical trials that collect a small amount of data from a large sample are the reverse of crossover and other designs that employ small samples. Which way to go depends on the purpose of the study as well as the outcomes to be measured. A large sample is useful in reducing the time in which outcomes can be assessed by increasing the power of the tests: an outcome such as occurrence of death is more likely to be observed in the larger sample. The advantage of larger samples is less important when outcomes can occur in a short time period, as they often do in evaluations of the nursing process. Moreover, large, simple trials are not necessarily inexpensive. The digoxin trial cost over $16 million.

Deviations From Ideal

With the appearance of large, simple trials on the research design scene, there is encouragement to explore simplification of research designs in general. Simplicity should be the byword, as the attempt is made to reduce costs of conducting research and speed up acquisition of findings. One way of achieving this is to maintain flexibility in using any type of research design, not just the RCT. This does *not* mean that standards for validity and reliability should be lowered. What is advocated is not to become a slave to the research process without careful regard for the study objectives, the likely findings, and their dissemination and utilization. An important question is: How much error can be tolerated? If highly precise findings are not necessary, greater freedom from rigid design principles is permissible.

Data Collection/Processing

Indirect, Projective and Proxy Data

There is a tendency, in constructing measures of variables for studies, to approach the task literally. If, for example, the study calls for a measure of the construct "quality of life," the usual approach is to define it directly as a combination of literal subvariables such as functional status, self-perceived health status, satisfaction with life, and negative and positive mood. Gathering data on such a complex variable requires a considerable measurement effort with associated problems of validity and reliability.

It might well be that other, perhaps less direct, measures could be found that would not only require easier data collection, but would be better indicators of quality of life; perhaps something as simple as the amount of time a person spends vacationing during a year. Perhaps a projective technique similar to the Rorschach test could obtain useful data on quality of life.

The term "proxy" refers to use of a substitute for the real thing. Proxy measures play an important role in research where it is difficult if not impossible to measure the literal construct. An excellent illustration of a proxy measure is provided by the investigation of the relationship between cholesterol and coronary heart disease (Consensus Development Conference, 1985). An early study examined the relationship between the cholesterol level of blood and deaths from atherosclerosis. Needless to say, the study took many years to complete and was very costly. Later studies used data obtained from arteriograms showing the thickness of fatty deposits on artery walls (from cholesterol) as a proxy for the outcome measure "deaths from atherosclerosis," because on autopsy a high correlation is found between size of the arterial channel and deaths.

Most clinical, physiologic, or laboratory measures are indirect or proxy measures or both. Body temperature is used as a proxy for general health status. We say that a person is sick if there is an elevated temperature. Similarly, a person's body weight, skin color, and respiration rate are used as proxies for measuring certain aspects of health status. There are also many indirect and proxy measures of sociopsychological and behavioral characteristics, such as creativity, emotional status, and personality, that are widely used in nursing studies.

Use of Secondary Data

Secondary data can have many uses in research. As has already been shown, they can substitute for the control group in clinical trials. They can also be helpful in planning a study, providing information useful to the formulation of the theoretical framework for the study, defining variables, designing data collection instruments, and analyzing and interpreting data.

The technique of meta-analysis takes secondary data to their ultimate productive use: They are the entire source of data for the study. For meta-analysis to work, a good supply of replicated or at least similar studies is needed as well as a computerized information system for storing and retrieving relevant data. Another beneficial source of data is found in the many different computerized record systems, such as the Medicare and Medicaid patient systems, with, of course, proper safeguards for privacy (Grady & Schwartz, 1993). Nursing is in the early stages of using such databases, but by the next century database analyses should be common practice in nursing research. McCormick (1992) has shown the potential value of existing databases in conducting effectiveness research in her inventory of nearly 100 federal, public, and private databases in the health field.

Cross Design Synthesis

Database analyses of records, aided by computer technology, can complement meta-analyses of completed studies. In fact, a merger of database and meta-analyses has been proposed (U. S. General Accounting Office, 1992). This would make the best use of both techniques by enlarging the pool of data available for analysis. Known as *cross design synthesis*, the method reduces the strict study selection requirements of meta-analysis by drawing upon different kinds of studies as well as compilations of statistical data from secondary sources. The major technical challenge is the need to adjust for imbalances in the comparison groups.

Synthesis of data from varied sources produces a study population with greater power than do replicated or similarly designed studies alone. This procedure is especially valuable in nursing research because diverse methods are often applied to the study of the same problem. Early application of this technique to evaluation of medical effectiveness holds promise for its usefulness in other areas of research.

Minimalist Approach

Some of the best studies have included small samples of study subjects and have relied on a bare minimum of statistical techniques. The ultimate minimalist design includes as few as one subject (Johannessen & Fosstvedt, 1991; Raymond, 1986). Piling up a large mass of quantitative data does not automatically yield better findings. A qualitative approach, using small samples and devoid of any statistics at all, can produce a rich understanding of the content and context of the area under study. As Jennings (1991) suggests, qualitative methods can help capture the reality of patient outcomes from an inductive perspective and provide a clearer sense of the dynamics of outcomes. Moreover, it is possible to advance the state of knowledge without conducting a research project at all. Computer-assisted techniques such as simulation can substitute for research in the quest for certain solutions to problems (Valinsky, 1975).

174 • NURSING RESEARCH METHODOLOGIES

Simplifying Data Collection

In collecting data most nursing studies use the traditional approaches of direct observation, mailed questionnaires, and interviews of either randomly or purposively selected study subjects. Other techniques are available that could possibly be more productive.

For example, there are techniques used by survey researchers in which data are collected by telephone or by recording instruments, such as monitors attached to television sets, to study viewership. A few nursing studies have employed television monitors to observe study subjects, or used physiologic monitors attached to subjects to make continuous recordings.

Another technique is use of a panel of subjects as a data source. A panel is different from a treatment or control group in that they are not subjected to an intervention, but are used as a continuing source of "natural state" information. Some longitudinal studies have used large groups of subjects as cohorts for collecting lifestyle data and clinical measurements (Kannel et al., 1986; Martin, Hulley, Browner, Kuller, & Wentworth, 1986).

In the future, advances in computer technology will make possible significant improvements in the speed and ease of collecting and analyzing research data. Interactive video, for example, will enable collection of large amounts of data on a wide variety of sociopsychological, economic, demographic, attitudinal, and behavioral variables almost overnight. This technology, coupled with super-speedy data processing, will make it possible to conduct a research project from beginning to end in a matter of days, instead of the months or even years that it now takes. Hand-held computers will also help speed up data collection and analysis. The Federal High Performance Computing and Communication (HPCC) Program will accelerate the availability and use of future high performance computers and networks (Office of Science and Technology Policy, 1992).

Data Analysis and Interpretation

Maximizing the Analytical Use of Data

Computers have made it easy to run and rerun multiple tabulations of data and statistical tests of the most esoteric kind. This is not what is meant by making the best use of data. What *is* meant is making the most *meaningful* use. Often, great scientific advances have been made with intensive rather than extensive analysis. Einstein's theory of relativity, after all, is expressed in a simple equation containing three clearly defined variables.

Using Simplified Techniques of Analysis

One shortcoming of some research textbooks is that they do not provide guidance on simple and meaningful alternative approaches to data analysis. Textbooks seem to be biased towards the use of more elaborate techniques and provide little practical direction to the researcher. The typical perspective of these books is that all techniques are important, advice is not offered on which could be the most efficient for the data at hand.

Sometimes it appears that a more complicated analytical approach is taken when a simpler one would do simply because it provides an impressive gloss to the data. As already mentioned, high-powered techniques such as analysis of variance and multiple regression are often applied to data when all the assumptions for their use have not been met. Depending on the data, a nonparametric technique may not only conveniently sidestep the restrictive assumptions, but may yield an equal amount of useful information. And, when a parametric technique is used, confidence intervals may be simpler to compute and to understand, yet be as informative as tests of significance.

Thinking Positively

Many research questions and hypotheses address only the negative side of the issue, focusing on why undesirable things occur. Researchers have until recently only studied causes of sickness and death and not "causes" of wellness. The search for the causes of breast cancer, for example, has generated many studies on lifestyle and heredity factors. Accompanying the recent interest in wellness has been a shift towards greater concern with positive health. Thus, research questions have progressed from what *causes* breast cancer, to what *prevents* breast cancer, to why is it that the majority of women, fortunately, will not develop breast cancer? In another research area, it is possible that more can be learned about job satisfaction by studying nurses who have stable employment histories than by studying those who move from one job to another. Finally, the question should not only be formulated in terms of why people have automobile accidents, but why it is that so many people avoid accidents—an amazing phenomenon considering the large numbers of today's bad drivers, bad roads, and bad vehicles.

Disseminating Research Findings

It is likely that at the present time a large store of useful research findings exists that has not had an impact on nursing practice. One reason is a resistance to change, as according to Hunt (1981), nursing is very traditional, ritualistic, and hierarchical. By the 21st century, an innovative and flexible style will hopefully pervade the practice of nursing and "research findings will provide indicators for practice and practice will provide new questions and problems for research. Nurses cannot, and should not, wait for some perfect solution" (Hunt, 1981, p. 184).

PART III

The Impact of Nursing Research on Society

Chapter 11

Nursing Research and Health Policy

Preparing for nursing research in the 21st century will require major shifts in our thinking. Researchers will no longer have the luxury of doing what they please. The federal dollar will flow toward programs that attack *society's* problems. Although basic science is important, many feel that too much is being spent on the search for new knowledge and not enough on harnessing the knowledge already gained. The emphasis is now on directed research to meet social needs (Donley, 1985). Science will be driven more by its consumers than by its products.

The challenge ahead for nurse researchers is to determine how best to use limited research dollars to develop new knowledge and to use that knowledge to solve society's problems. At the National Institutes of Health (NIH)—the mecca for medical research—scientists have had to redefine their roles and recognize that the mission of NIH is *not* to serve the scientists, but the needs of the public.

Increasing numbers of nurse researchers are now emphasizing the importance of the linkage between clinical practice and research (Moritz, 1991). Questions relevant to improving clinical practice must first be asked and then answered. Studies directed by nurses, as well as those in which they collaborate with others, can discover better and cheaper care for patients.

Up to now, the growth in nursing research has not been paralleled by a comparable growth in the use of research findings in clinical practice nor in impact on health care policy decisions.

Most health professionals and congressional leaders agree that the health care system is "our sickest patient." It is encouraging that more than 40 nursing organizations have joined forces in drafting a nursing agenda for health reform (Nurses Propose Health Care Reform, 1991; Plan Calls for Health Care Reform, 1991). The agenda emphasizes a system that promotes primary health care and the promotion, restoration, and maintenance of health for all Americans (Johnson, 1993). A focus on managed competition will attempt to control runaway inflation through cost-effective delivery of health care. Managed competition is a way of organizing choices under both employment-based and publicly financed insurance programs (Starr, 1992).

As emphasis is placed on quality improvement based on outcomes, nurse researchers will be involved in measurements at the bedside that will help to document the most effective systems of health care delivery. Johnson (1993) states that assessment of health care needs must be the determining factor in structuring and delivering health care programs and services. Most of all, nurses must work in partnership with consumers.

> Information on quality is absolutely critical. This was reinforced by Richard I. Smith, former Public Policy Director, Washington Business Group on Health where he emphasized that the real revolution that is going to occur in health care reform is accountability. (Washington Post January 1, 1993)

Nursing Research and Health Policy Decisionmaking

Nurse researchers are in a unique position to make special contributions to health policy analysis. They can help policymakers make more informed choices if they can make their voices heard (Abdellah, 1991). The settings and sites in which nurses function enable them to identify the potential health consequences of policies, and to bring these consequences to the attention of those guiding policies. Nurses can formulate and identify questions for policy research and policy analysis; for example, questions related to child abuse and elder abuse, and questions raised about reporting and confidentiality. The front line situations occupied by nurses make them most able to identify and measure cost benefits, quality of care, outcomes, and underlying ethical issues related to practice. Nurse researchers need to take advantage of their position and articulate the issues based on theoretical, practical, and applied knowledge.

The research process is highly pertinent to policy formulations if the findings can be shown to have a significant impact on nursing practice.

> Good policy analysis demands the application of research; therefore, the scientific community, and especially nursing, should give more attention to the role research can play in policy formulation. Policy analysis is NOT concerned with new knowledge development but with summarizing the best available information that is related to the choices among policy alternatives. (Kessler, 1989, p. 246)

For research findings to be useful to policymakers, they must be relevant to real world problems and provide options that contribute to the resolution of the problems. Nurse researchers have an obligation to present their findings in such a way that they can be considered in the policy process.

In the past, nursing research has had a significant impact on policy. The classic study of the Committee for the Study of Nursing Education (Committee for the Study of Nursing Education, 1923) initiated a number of major changes in the organization and operations of schools of nursing in the United States, some of which changes are still being implemented. The time and motion studies of nursing activities, begun in the 1930s under the auspices of the National League for Nursing Education (now NLN), resulted in major changes in the ways in which nursing services were delivered. The Progressive Patient Care Study, conducted in the late 1950s had a major impact on how patient care was organized, the most notable example being the growth of intensive care units and the evolvement of nursing specialties such as critical care nurses (Abdellah & Levine, 1986).

Thus, clinical nursing research is beginning to make an impact. An example is the research on urinary incontinence in adults that documents a connection between the findings related to nursing practices and needed changes in health policies.

To understand the importance of nursing research to society in shaping the health agenda and restructuring the health care system, the meaning of public health policy must be clarified.

Public Health Policy Defined

Public health policy formulation is the way issues are raised on the public agenda; the process by which laws are passed committing resources to programs that affect people; the development or withdrawal of rules and regulations that interpret laws; the process of program implementation; and the evaluation of the usefulness of the program to improving practice through nursing research (Aiken, 1982).

The definitions of policy and politics are interrelated. Policy is referred to as a plan of action, a way of management, practical wisdom and prudence, and political skill. Policy implies "for the public good" and is both benevolent and utilitarian. Politics is often referred to as the art of science of government concerned with guiding or influencing health policy.

Types of research related to health policy are as follows:

Policy Research

This is an empirical investigation of the application of a policy to uncover its effects. The scope is limited, usually focused on past events, and uses primary data rather than relying on subjective judgments. One example is the inclusion of women as study subjects in studies of the causes of fetal alcoholism or cholesterol-related heart disease. Previous research had not considered women in relation to their health problems even though heart disease is a leading cause of death in women.

Evaluation Research

This research tests outcomes of alternative policies. This research can be either retrospective or prospective. Research methods used in policy research include:

- Compilation of previous research;
- Surveys (demographic, epidemiological, public opinion, historical);
- Cost-benefit and risk-benefit analysis;
- Operation research techniques;
- Systems analysis;
- Simulation;

- Trend extrapolation;
- Field investigation; and
- Use of expert panels, for example, Delphi techniques.

Disciplinary Research

This is focused on developing and testing theories in a specific area that may or may not be useful for policymakers. Research findings that are not translated into terms that policymakers can understand will garner scant attention and have little impact on future health policy.

A good example is Brooten's (1986) research of low-birth weight infants, which goes beyond theory to document quality of care and cost savings (See Chapter 6, pp. 74–75).

The Federal Government's Role in Health Policy Formulation

Why is there a growing interest in public policy? The rapid escalation of federal health expenditures since 1965 has forced health policy into the political arena and into public consciousness (Figure 11.1). Federal health expenditures have grown from $3 billion a year in 1960 to $800 billion in 1992—12% of the U. S. gross national product (GNP)—yet 37 million Americans have no access to health care or are underinsured and the numbers in both categories are rapidly growing. By the year 2000, the cost of medical benefits will exceed $22,000 per worker (Benson, 1991), and as yet, the public has not been offered solutions to the problem.

Where does the $800 billion go (Figure 11.2)? The federal government finances, through federal taxes, well over one-third of all medical expenditures in the United States, mostly through direct financing programs. Presently, the federal government's complex array of health programs falls into four categories:

1. Direct care programs for some populations either directly (e.g., Department of Defense, Indian Health Service, Department of Veterans Affairs) or through grant programs such as the Women, Infants, and Children (WIC) program.
2. Federal programs to pay for medical care services—Medicare and Medicaid, as well as federal employees' health benefits programs and programs for the military and their dependents.

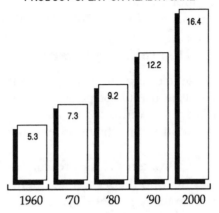

PERCENTAGE OF U.S. GROSS NATIONAL
PRODUCT SPENT ON HEALTH CARE

SOURCE: Health Care Financing Administration

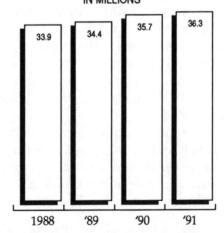

NUMBER OF NONELDERLY AMERICANS
WITHOUT HEALTH COVERAGE,
IN MILLIONS

SOURCE: Employee Benefit Research Institute
tabulations of the Current Population Survey,
March '89, '90, '91, '92

Figure 11.1   The cost of health care in the year 2000 versus the recent
number of elderly Americans without health care coverage.
Washington Post Health/January 26, 1993.

3. Programs designed to regulate the supply of medical resources to improve the quality of services, for example, Medicare regulations regarding nursing homes that require minimum safety standards and quality of care.
4. Programs to fund medical research or public health activities (e.g., immunizations) (Arras, 1981).

How Federal Policy Affects Health Care Providers

Health care providers have become increasingly interested in public policy, particularly federal health policy, as it directly affects their own interests. The professional activities of health providers are greatly influenced by federal policies and programs. There are, however, limitations as to what these policies can do. This must be understood so that energies can be directed towards implementing strategies that will accomplish stated goals, whatever they might be. Health providers must take care not to overestimate the capacity of the federal government to affect practice (Cohn, 1992).

Policy decisions made by industry often have a greater impact on nursing practice, especially in the areas of health insurance payment, than do the public health policy decisions of the federal government. However, there are four ways in which federal health policies affect health care providers:

- The federal government pays for health care for the poor, elderly, and disabled;
- Federal health manpower programs support the training of health care providers to influence the supply, composition, or distribution of the work force;
- Federally supported research provides the source for new ideas, innovations, and technical assistance; and
- Federal programs provide capital support for new and renovated health care facilities.

The Need for Health Care Reform

The present arrangement of health care delivery is under scrutiny. The potential for change is so high that nursing leaders cannot afford to ignore policies that deny health care to millions of Americans (Davis, 1993; Smith, 1988).

How does a nation of 250 million people spend $800 billion on health care each year?
Here's how, according to the latest estimates from the Department of Health and Human Services:

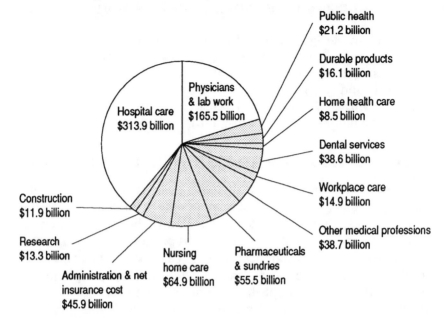

Public health
$21.2 billion

Durable products
$16.1 billion

Home health care
$8.5 billion

Dental services
$38.6 billion

Workplace care
$14.9 billion

Other medical professions
$38.7 billion

Physicians & lab work
$165.5 billion

Hospital care
$313.9 billion

Construction
$11.9 billion

Research
$13.3 billion

Administration & net insurance cost
$45.9 billion

Nursing home care
$64.9 billion

Pharmaceuticals & sundries
$55.5 billion

Hospital care—$313.9 billion. Includes spending on everything that happens inside the walls of the nation's 6,000-plus hospitals each year, including all inpatient and outpatient care, treatment by physicians and prescriptions dispensed, as well as hospital-based home nursing care.

Physician and laboratory services—$165.5 billion. This money goes to the doctors in private and group practice, the salaries of others who work for health maintenance organizations (HMOs) and laboratory fees.

Dental services—$38.6 billion. Money spent each year on visits to private practice dentists, on dental laboratory work and on the salaries for dentists who work for HMOs.

Other medical professionals—$38.7 billion. Includes the salaries of health care personnel other than physicians and dentists, such as private-duty nurses, chiropractors, podiatrists, speech and occupational therapists, midwives and optometrists.

Home health care—$8.5 billion. Accounts for skilled nurses and other personnel and services for homebound patients. It includes information from Medicare cost reports filed by Medicare-certified home health agencies, which covers only a portion of all the people who receive medical care at home.

Pharmaceuticals and sundries—$55.5 billion. Retail sales amount spent each year on prescription drugs including items such as bandages and nonprescription drugs.

Durable products—$16.1 billion. Expenditures for eyeglasses, contact lenses, hearing aids, wheelchairs and artificial limbs.

Nursing home care—$64.9 billion. Inpatient nursing and personal care facilities.

Workplace care—$14.9 billion. Medical care provided by industrial employers at or near the workplace.

Administration of government health programs and the net cost of health insurance—$45.9 billion. Includes three components. The largest part is the difference between what insurance companies take in as premiums from subscribers and what they pay to hospitals, doctors, and other care givers in benefits. That difference, which is included here, could be a company's profit, shareholders' dividends, the reserves an insurer must have, and commisions to insurance agents. The second-largest part is the expense of administering government health programs, the largest of which are Medicaid, Medicare and the health services of the Defense and Veterans Affairs departments. The third component is the administrative expenses of nongovernmental philanthropic organizations, such as the grant-writing, fund-raising and administrative costs of the American Red Cross or the American Cancer Society.

Public health—$21.2 billion. This money is spent by the federal government mainly to operate the Centers for Disease Control and the Food and Drug Administration. Also, funding for state and local government health departments.

Research—$13.3 billion. Medical and health care research done by nonprofit or government entities accounts for this figure. Drug research undertaken by drug manufacturers is not included.

Construction—$11.9 billion. This sum equals the cost of constructing hospitals and nursing homes plus additions, alterations and major renovations.

SOURCE: Department of Health and Human Services

Figure 11.2 An $800 billion health care bill—where it went in 1992.

Three areas key to health care reform are: access to care, quality of care, and reduced costs. Improvements in these areas may make up the paradigm to the solution of the health care crisis. Nurse researchers must be willing to be part of this solution by utilizing research and practice to identify outcomes linked to quality care. This will help to assure the maximum cost-effective use of resources (Kos-Munson, 1993).

Thus, theory building and health policymaking must be embedded in the needs of society. The mandate seems clear. We need a system that is focused on prevention, health maintenance, and the integration and coordination of care; a system that yields the greatest output in the most user-friendly way (Bentley, 1992).

The Problem of Health Care Access

Access to care is a problem of increasing magnitude. It is in large measure dependent upon health insurance to pay the fee for the service; those lacking health insurance can only go to the emergency room for care. The highest rates of uninsured are found among young adults, blacks, Hispanics, and in families where no one is employed, but increasingly, middle-class families are falling into this category.

Nurse researchers have not adequately shown a linkage between nursing research and access to care. Theory, research, and practice must be an integral part of *access*. Stevens (1993) cautions that access must be a focal element of theory, research, and practice as it affects policy decisions determining the availability of health care. Stevens suggests that to integrate equitable access to health care as a research goal, nurse researchers need to go beyond conceptualizing at the individual level and instead theoretically frame access in its broadest sociopolitical context

Nurses gather data that would be useful to health policy decision-makers regarding access to health care. Nurses must systematically document the nature and frequency of barriers to health care. Health care initiatives supported by quantitative data can be more effective in influencing health policy decisions. (Bonuck & Avno, 1993).

The debate on how individuals shall have access to available care raises the following questions: (Williams, 1986)

1. Who shall decide which persons receive minimal care or the full array of services?

2. What kind of services will be provided, and what shall be the quality and quantity of these services?
3. Who shall decide which health care providers will perform which functions? Who will implement and enforce the policies? Who will receive direct reimbursement for services provided?
4. Will nurses participate in the policy decisionmaking process?

Today, and into the future, the emphasis on disease prevention and health promotion should be increased. Williams (1986) recognizes the importance of nurses in communicating values to their patients/clients.

Would planned governmental rationing of health care work? It might if all available health care resources were being utilized efficiently, which is not happening. A better approach would be to eliminate wasteful practices. The Medical Treatment Effectiveness Program of the Agency for Health Care Policy and Research (AHCPR)—discussed in greater detail on pp. 204–5—is a better approach than rationing of medical care.

AHCPR is attempting to learn the effects of current medical and nursing practices on patients' survival and quality of life. By identifying the most effective treatments and providing this information to health care providers and policymakers, there is the potential for improving care and controlling health care costs at the same time.

Defining Health Problems in Terms of Policy Issues

Health problems must be defined in terms of health policy issues. Health became firmly embedded in the political agenda in 1979 with the release of the first *Surgeon General's Report on Health Promotion and Disease Prevention*, which called for a national health strategy to emphasize the prevention of disease. Scientific knowledge alone does not solve major health problems. Personal discipline and political will are also essential (Milio, 1984). The individual, can do more for his or her own health and well-being than any doctor, any hospital, any drug, any exotic medical device. Even when aware that health practices are detrimental to one's health, individuals may cling to old habits. Altering one's lifestyle is not easy even when a person is well motivated.

"It is the controllability of many risks—and,often the significance of controlling even only a few—that lies at the heart of disease prevention and health promotion." (U. S. Department of Health Education and Welfare, p. 13, 1979)

Health policy is any policy that influences the health of the population. Thus, public policy can serve as a guide to government action (e.g., by legislation, executive order, or regulatory mandate). Examples of social issues that have impact on the delivery of health services and policy formulation are the need to provide quality and compassionate care for the homeless, the elderly, the chronically ill, and people with AIDS. These issues comprise a major portion of the public agenda and are reinforced by the American Nurses Association, (ANA) agenda for health policy reform (American Nurses Association [ANA], 1989).

ANA's Agenda for Health Care Reform

The American Nurses Association has drafted "Nursing's Agenda for Health Care Reform (American Nurses Association, 1989, 1992), to summarize the nursing profession's position in the health care reform debate and to stimulate action. The major areas of emphasis in this plan are as follows:

Essential Elements of the ANA Plan

- A restructured health care system that enhances consumer access to health care;
- A federally defined standard package of essential health care services available to all citizens, financed through private and public plans;
- Funding of basic needs, for example, needs of women, infants, and children; housing and energy assistance for the poor, the elderly, and mentally ill; clean air and clean water; and occupational safety and health;
- Privacy health care including direct reimbursement of nurse practitioners;
- Steps to reduce health care costs, such as required use of managed care;
- Case management required;

- Attention to human rights;
- Nursing research and education;
- Access to services assured; and
- Public/private sector review (American Nurses Association, 1991).

Managed Care: Can it Work? (As Referred to in ANA Plan)

Managed care currently exists in two forms. One is case-by-case review and approvals and denials in traditional insurance coverage. The other is enrollment in health maintenance organizations (HMOs) or plans such as Kaiser Permanente. Managed care has had some success. There have also been some problems, such as risk sharing among doctors who decide if patients should be referred to specialists or undergo expensive tests. Managed care can also protect patients from ineffective therapies (Cohn, 1992). For example, clinical practice guidelines, such as those published by the Agency for Health Care Policy and Research, can help health care providers to avoid ineffective therapies.

Primary Health Care (ANA Plan)

Primary health care is characterized as an array of health care services that are accessible and acceptable to the patient, comprehensive in scope, coordinated and continuous over time, and for which the practitioner is accountable for the quality of services provided (Nutting, 1991).Primary health care practitioners interact with ambulatory patients/clients at the initial contact between the individual and the health care system. Primary health care—an essential element in any health care plan—provides an integrating function, balancing the multiple requirements of patient/client problems. The practitioner uses information developed from many sources to develop a strategy for optional resolution of the patient's/client's condition.

Primary health care has strong consumer involvement and becomes important in health policy formulation and involvement of health practitioners in decision making. Health policy reform also includes a major emphasis on health promotion and disease prevention. Murphy (1992) links the principles of primary health care to responsive and flexible health care services that influence health policy decision making.

Strengthening Nursing's Role in Health Policy Formulation

There is increasing involvement of nursing leaders in health policy—but the focus is obfuscated by placing the emphasis on issues affecting nursing as a profession rather than on health issues (Pender, 1992a). Nurse researchers seldom identify the policy implications of their research and may not be aware of the issues. Milio (1984) suggests that if nurses are serious about influencing health policy, policy must be seen as process rather than content. Policy is NOT static. Milio points out that policy formulation is shaped by the social and political process that forms it.

Nurses must become active players in the process of health policy formulation (Smith, 1988). The allocation of health care resources and decisions about who will receive these resources must involve nurses, otherwise nursing will be forced to deal with problems in retrospect rather than prospectively (Rooks, 1990).

Nurse faculty need to encourage students to identify the policy implications of their research. Clinical placement of students in policy-oriented settings is essential, for example, placement as a Congressional fellow working with Congressional staffers in the formulation of health policies. Senator Daniel K. Inouye (D-HI) has championed this approach for many years and utilized nurse Congressional fellows on his staff. Another example is the "Nurses in Washington Roundtable" sponsored by nurses in health policy positions in the Washington, DC, area.

Doctoral students must be encouraged to pursue research oriented to political and social realities. Nurses need to disseminate general health services and health systems information to policymakers, decisionmakers, and consumers.

At the University of Pittsburgh School of Nursing, a specific doctoral level course has been added to the curriculum focusing on nursing leadership and public policy. Doctoral students examine the role of nursing as a major health care provider in professional, social, and political contexts; evaluate landmark pieces of legislation in terms of economic, ethical, social, cultural, and political factors; identify the leadership role in shaping public policies; and develop the skills needed in health policy development (Martin, White & Hansen, 1989).

There is a valid role for the nurse in health care management at the policymaking level. Health policies often fail because of opposition from those whose responsibility it is to implement them, who had little or no input into their development. The broader the base of input, the closer to reality will be the end product, and the greater will be the cooperation and enthusiasm of the implementors (Rice, 1987).

The process of policymaking must involve all levels of the organizational structure. It cannot be isolated, but instead be a "reflective process," ongoing and continuously being reviewed to meet the changing times. Any policy decision will affect some segment of society. Health policy decisions often affect the most vulnerable in our society—the handicapped, the elderly, the mentally ill, minorities, and those with AIDS. Nurses have a responsibility to participate fully in policymaking. As the caring profession, it is to the nurse that the patient/client turns for help.

Nurses Can Affect Policy Formulation at Three Levels

- The individual patient,
- The practice environment, and
- National policy (Hinshaw, 1988).

To influence health policy, nurses must seek the widest, most knowledgeable audience for their research findings. This means publishing beyond scientific journals and also in clinical practice and administrative journals. Brooten and Martinson are excellent examples (Brooten et al., 1986; Martinson, 1981). For example, Brooten published her research in the *New England Journal of Medicine*, documenting care and costs of low-birthweight infants.

Hinshaw (1988b) suggests that research findings be synthesized with societal needs and professional priorities, for example, as defining and structuring nursing research; identifying high-priority research issues, both societal and professional; and identifying specific research findings ready for application.

In their review of nurse-midwifery research, Diers and Burst (1983) state that health policy of this specialty group has evolved largely from the use of data from evaluation studies. Such data include infant and maternal mortality rates, birthweights, and cost-effective figures—basic outcome statistics that substantiated the value of these practitioners. Diers and Burst emphasizes that research findings need to be kept simple and understandable to have impact on policy.

Nursing Values and Health Care Policy

The decade of the '90s and the coming 21st century will bring a return to a more value-centered world (Naisbitt & Aburdene 1990). The problems of the homeless, AIDS, and drug use will continue to move health care into the forefront, demanding changes of priorities in health policies. Cost containment will continue as a policy issue and will be more closely linked with quality (Maraldo, 1990). Consumers will become more vocal about their health concerns as access to health care becomes more difficult. The efforts of organized nursing to seek direct reimbursement for nursing services under Medicare will place nursing in greater prominence, allowing the profession more input into how health policies affecting the allocation of resources should be optimally allocated to best serve the patient/client. As the population ages, increased demand for care of those with chronic illness will lead to emphasis upon managed care and the pivotal role of nurse practitioner as its provider.

Values give direction to policy development. Therefore, as nurses delineate their own values, they can serve as a guide to influencing public policy, particularly health care policy. Davis (1988) suggests a "values-policy model" as one approach to evaluating the effect of values on policy (Figure 11.3). The model has four phases:

Phase I: Values are standards and patterns of choice that guide policy direction.

Phase II: Serves as the bridge to public policy based on input of data and information that influences the outcomes.

Phase III: Social and health policy become official through law and regulations.

Phase IV: Policy evaluated by impact on social and economic policy.

The issues that society elects to confront set priorities on the national health agenda. Some issues, such as AIDS, are of such magnitude that they are thrust upon the public consciousness, but others equally important, such as proper nutrition and healthy lifestyles, receive less attention.

In ANA's *Nursing: A Social Statement*, the following concerns are integral to the formulation of social and health policies (American Nurses Association, 1980).

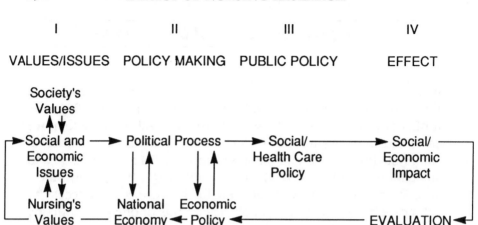

Source: Davis, G. C. (1988). Nursing Values and Health Care Policy. *Nursing Outlook, 36,* 289–292.

Figure 11.3 The values-policy model.

- Belief in the individual's right to health care;
- Belief in humanistic health care;
- Belief in the individual's responsibility for his or her own health care; and
- Belief in the provision of health care by the best qualified practitioner.

Types of Health Policy Research: Five Broad National Goals

Types of health policy are government-commissioned policy analysis research, program evaluation policy research, and theoretical or experimental disciplinary research with policy implications as defined earlier.

Research undertaken for policy development purposes must be translated into terms readily understood by its intended audience, or it will not gain the support necessary to bring about action. It must focus attention on the implications of the findings for policy development in specific settings (policy research) or their use in a broader sense (policy analysis).

Five broad national goals for the year 2000 that affect health policy formulation are listed below:

By the Year 2000. . .

1. Reduce infant mortality to no more than 7 deaths per 1,000 live births.
2. Increase life expectancy to at least 78 years.
3. Reduce disability caused by chronic conditions to a prevalence of no more than 7.0 percent of all people.
4. Increase healthy years of life to at least 65 years.
5. Decrease disparity in life expectancy between white and minority populations to no more than 4 years (U. S. Department of Health and Human Services, 1991).

1.   Reduce Infant Mortality to No More Than 7 Deaths per 1,000 Live Births

The infant mortality rate traditionally has been considered one of the best overall indicators of a nation's health—and of a nation's commitment to ensuring the health of its people. It is a commonly used indicator for international comparisons.

For the past two decades, the United States' infant mortality rate has declined steadily, reaching 10.4 percent per 1,000 live births in 1986, and 9.6 in 1991, the lowest infant mortality rate ever recorded in the United States.

The decline in infant mortality during the 1970s is attributable largely to a marked reduction in mortality among low-birthweight infants as a result of advances in neonatal intensive care and dissemination of information to the health community and the general public. There was a small improvement in the birthweight distribution during the 1970s, but during the 1980s the birthweight distribution remained essentially constant. Success in attaining the year 2000 target will require further improvement in the birthweight distribution. Nurse practitioners, and particularly nurse-midwives, can help to achieve this goal. Programs targeted to high-risk groups need to be generated and vigorously pursued by health care givers, because attention paid to these groups will eventually pay off by lowering health care costs.

Infant mortality rates vary substantially among and within racial/ ethnic groups. The relatively low national rate of 10.3 hides the radical differences among American Indian communities, some of which have infant mortality rates approaching twice the national rate. The rate for black infants (18.0) continues to be twice that of white infants (8.9).

According to international rankings of infant mortality rates, the United States ranked 20th in infant mortality in 1984 and 19th in 1985! This poor international ranking of a country of great wealth and social sophistication is of great concern to health activists and an area in which much progress still needs to be made.

2. Increase Life Expectancy From 75 Years to at Least 78 Years

Life expectancy at birth, the number of years an individual is expected to live, is another important measure of a nation's health. It also is a standard measure for international comparisons and summarizes a population's current mortality experience in terms of average survival.

3. Reduce Disability Caused by Chronic Conditions to a Prevalence of No More Than 7.0%

Disability caused by chronic conditions is defined as a limitation in major activity because of chronic conditions. "Major activity" refers to the usual activity for one's age-sex group, whether it is working, keeping house, going to school, or living independently. Chronic conditions are defined as conditions that either were first noticed 3 or more months ago or which belong to a group of conditions, such as heart disease and diabetes, which are considered chronic regardless of time of origin.

The fact that life expectancy is high does not indicate whether the population is predominantly well or is heavily burdened with chronic illness and disability. In 1987, 8.9% of the population suffered a limitation in major activity due to chronic conditions. About 3.7% were unable to carry on a major activity, and an additional 5.2% were limited in the amount or kind of major activity they could perform.

In 1991, an Institute of Medicine study reported that 35 million Americans suffer from physical and metal disabilities at an annual cost of $110 billion (Rich, 1991). The target set for the year 2000 of 7.0% would represent more than a 20% reduction in disability due to chronic conditions between 1987 and the year 2000. This situation will require long-term planning and emphasis on health promotion and disease prevention to change lifestyles and prevent disabilities.

4. Increase Healthy Years of Life to at Least 65 Years

Healthy years of life (also referred to as quality-adjusted life years) is defined as the duration or quantity of life discounted by some estimate of the quality of life. It is a summary measure of health that combines mortality (quantity of life) and morbidity (quality of life) into a single measure. Like life expectancy, it reflects the situation of all age groups.

In recent years, considerable research effort has been devoted to developing a health status index, a comprehensive measure of the health of the population. Although several approaches have been developed for combining mortality and morbidity, the quality-adjusted life year (QALY) is a commonly used health status measure. The goal for the year 2000 is to increase years of healthy life by 5 years, from 60 to 65.

The impact of health policies on health services delivery of care to the elderly is already evident today, as public policymakers grapple with the difficult problem of financing long-term care services in the future. Long-term (LTC) care may very well be the major public issue of the next decade because there is an ever-increasing demand for this type of care. Demand for publicly supported LTC services is already estimated to be three times greater than supply and will increase rapidly as the population ages. The importance of rethinking national health policies and programs for the elderly with much more attention to ambulatory, home care and long-term care, as well as more cost controls, is long overdue. Long-term care regulation is cyclical in nature—disappointing provider performance resulting in new and tougher regulations, then in increased expectations and disillusionment when those expectations are not fulfilled. New health policies that improve health care delivery may change the roller coaster nature of long-term care regulations.

5. Decrease Disparity in Life Expectancy Between White and Minority Populations to No More Than 4 Years

According to the most recent census, members of racial and ethnic minority groups account for 20.1% of the U. S. population, including blacks (11.5%), Hispanics (6.4%), Asians/Pacific Islanders (1.5%), and American Indian/Alaska Natives (0.6%). In the year 2000, racial and ethnic minorities are expected to comprise about 25% of the population, with blacks and Hispanics accounting for about 13.1% and 11.6% respectively. Minority and disadvantaged communities lag behind the white U. S. population on virtually all health status indicators. Some of the problems involve access to care and low economic status, as well as social isolation, inferior education, and risky health behaviors.

The difficulties involved in bringing about health behavior change are addressed by Shumaker, Schron, and Ockene (1990) in relation to obstacles to life-style change and adherence. There are multiple factors that inhibit a person's ability to make changes in their lifestyle. Those most frequently identified are biological as well as psychological barriers to adoption and maintenance of health-promoting behaviors.

The goal as well as the challenge to health professionals is to view health strategies in a way so as to accept the social specification of optimal care, while at the same time safeguarding the individual practitioner's role as an advocate for each patient/client and the nursing profession's role as an advocate of its view of the public good and public policy. The mandate is the pursuit of efficiency and quality of care (Donabedian, 1988).

Data Needed for Policy Decisionmaking

Obtaining data for health policy research requires monitoring the course of events relevant to policy; forecasting emerging problems prior to their surfacing; identifying and analyzing problem-raising situations; critiquing current policies when based on lack of understanding; redefining a problem; and analyzing the policymaking process.

Nursing needs to face the fact that scientific data are very often not influential in policymaking and are not the type of information often used. What is needed are the kinds of information that are strategic and can answer the question: "How can policy proposal X be made feasible and effective?" (Milio, 1984). For example, the use of clinical practice guidelines by health practitioners can improve quality of care and may reduce costs.

Policy makers are seeking information (data) that will answer the following questions:

1. How to define policy problems in the context of health promotion, attitude change, and behavior modification, and how to gain the public's support;
2. How to select the most effective policy instruments to address priority health issues and how to promote the use of these instruments; and
3. How to develop strategies that will ensure effective implementation and adoption of these instruments.

In 1988, the Institute of Medicine of the National Academy of Sciences published the recommendation that health organizations become active in using a strategic approach to health-promoting policymaking (Institute of Medicine, 1988).

A committee recommended that every public health agency regularly and systematically collect, assemble, analyze, and make available information on the health of its client community. A plea was made that every public health agency responsibly serve the public interest in the development of comprehensive health policies by promoting use of scientific knowledge in public health decisionmaking. Needed data include statistics on health status, community health needs, and epidemiologic and other studies of health problems.

To meet the information needs of policymakers, new theoretical models and qualitative methods are necessary. Such methods rely on descriptive, observational data obtained from interviews, health hearings (both state and regional), content analyses of completed studies, and participant observation. The purpose is to understand and generate meaningful guidelines for the formulation of health policies.

Outcomes—Measures of Health Care Quality: The Key to Effective Health Policy Decisionmaking

Definitive data are needed for health policy decisionmaking. Findings of research can influence policy if the researcher provides the policymaker with explicit information as to how the findings can be used in improving clinical practice.

Because policy is a course of action that guides resource allocation, nurse leaders agree that a primary strategy for bringing about change is the use of data related to outcomes of nursing care. Researchers can influence health policy by providing information to guide and improve nursing practice.

What is needed are accurate databases drawn from systematic evaluation of nursing care interventions and innovative models, both administrative and clinical.

The measurement of outcomes has become centrally important to providing information for health policy makers. There is assiduous recognition of the importance of applying outcomes-oriented quality measurements in health care delivery. Outcomes measures, discussed in Chapter 7, refer to any measurement system used to uncover or identify the health outcome of treatment for the patient. Outcomes measurements now rely on easily defined elements such as mortality, morbidity, unnecessary hospital procedures, readmissions, and patient satisfaction. Many agree, however, that the ideal measure of quality is the patient's quality of life (Geigle & Jones, 1990).

The goals of outcomes measurement are viewed differently by the purchaser (who wants value for the health dollar), the provider (who wants the best care for the patient), and the patient (who wants to maintain or achieve a quality of life).

The next crucial need in relation to identifying outcomes measures is for reliable and useful data. There is heavy reliance on quantitative data and not enough on qualitative data. Why is it so difficult to identify qualitative data? There is lack of consensus as to how best to measure outcomes, that is, what tools are appropriate and what constitutes appropriate care. There is little evidence of the effectiveness and complication rates, on the quality of life effects from many medical treatments and procedures (Geigle & Jones 1990).

Consumers should be educated to become more conscious of variations in care and to demand quality care. Coordinated managed care and long-term care information could help to achieve the patient's goal of improved quality of life.

Quality of care, as well as cost effectiveness, are part of the decisionmaking process of health policy. For too long, patients/clients have been overlooked and uninvolved in determining outcomes measures that are linked to quality of care. Needed are:

- Patient opinions and data to evaluate the outcomes of an episode of care (patients can help to decide which treatments are best);
- Involvement of family and caregivers in determining outcome measures;
- Hospitals, long-term care, and home care programs which commit resources to quality of care;

- Nursing protocols for the treatment of selected diagnoses and conditions;
- Assurance that there is a true commitment at all levels to quality of care;
- Baseline data from many institutions and individuals; and
- Quality defined through data, surveys, algorithms, and the computer.

From the time of Florence Nightingale, efforts have been made to use patient outcomes to describe and measure nursing practice. Attempts to classify outcomes, however, are new (Agency for Health Care Policy and Research, 1991, 1992).

In 1980, the ANA issued *Nursing: A Social Policy Statement*, which defined four characteristics of nursing: phenomena, theory application, nursing action, and evaluation of effects in relation to phenomena. Six years later, the ANA Board of Directors approved the development of a classification system in which the key focus was the classification of assessment, diagnosis, interventions, and outcomes (Griffith, 1989). The classification system was to be used as a way to reach a consensus on a national basis to guide nursing information systems as well as health policy.

Historically, outcome measures are embedded in such classic works as Hasselmeyer's (1961) who studied the effects on premature infants of diaper roll support; and the work of Schwartz, Henley, & Zeitz (1964) who researched the nursing and psychosocial needs of the elderly ambulatory patient; Aydelotte (1962) who examined patient welfare as an outcome of nursing care; Abdellah and Levine (1957a) who developed a tool to measure patient satisfaction as a primary outcome measure of nursing care; Abdellah, Beland, Martin, & Matheney (1960) who developed an early classification system of 21 nursing problems that included assessment, nursing diagnosis, interventions, and outcomes; Hover and Zimmer (1978) who developed a quality assurance system that classified outcomes; and McCormick (1988) who looked at outcome measures in nursing homes in relation to incontinence.

As classification systems developed and placed emphasis on self-care and rehabilitation, one common factor emerged: Perception of patient care is a valuable outcome of care and research and researchers should continue to develop measures sensitive to patient satisfaction (Lang & Dorman, 1990). Data classification systems should be included in the development of national databases.

Data Needed

- Further research to measure specific aspects of nursing care and the determinants of satisfaction and the relationship between quality and satisfaction;
- More definitive evidence of process and outcome linkages;
- Data regarding the relationships between technology and assessment and quality assessment;
- Data regarding the reliability and validity of outcome measures as screening tools;
- Health status measures;
- Identification of specific "products" (outcomes) that will result from nursing efforts (Brooten, 1988; Fineberg, 1985).
- Sources of costs in the clinical area, both inpatient and outpatient;
- Data on the relationship between clinical judgment and administrative units in a hospital;
- Data on the cost and health consequences of clinical strategies;
- Data regarding patterns and variations in nurse behavior and behavior under payment patterns that offer strong levers of cost control;
- Development of prescribed guidelines by nurses and by other decisionmakers in the health care system;
- Identification of practice and reliable methods of assessment of quality;
- Determining cost of nursing services for DRGs using the acuity-of-illness-based method;
- Data that describe the relationships between nursing interventions and patient outcomes, with attention to cost effectiveness; and
- Data that describe nursing care in organized nursing services and that compare nurses with other health professionals in their effectiveness with patients in the cost of delivering services.

Outcomes measurements related to evaluation (effectiveness) of nurse practitioner practice can have considerable impact on policy and change research agendas. High on the health agenda are the health needs of special populations (minorities, the disabled, infants, and the elderly). Public policy that focuses on how to deliver services to these people offers special opportunities for nurse practitioners to provide data that demonstrates suitability, quality of care, and cost effectiveness (Molde and Diers, 1985).

Clinical Practice Guidelines

One effort to improve patient outcomes has been the development of clinical practice guidelines by the Agency for Health Care Policy and Research (AHCPR). This agency was established in December 1989 as the successor to the National Center for Health Services Research and Health Care Technology Assessment. AHCPR is one of nine agencies of the U. S. Public Health Service.

The Office of the Forum for Quality and Effectiveness in Health Care (AHCPR) develops and updates guidelines to be used in the management of clinical conditions. These guidelines are formulated as part of the Medical Treatment Effectiveness Program (MEDTEP), that also includes database development, effectiveness and outcomes research, and dissemination of research findings and guidelines.

The goal of AHCPR's dissemination of guidelines is to encourage health care providers to change their practice behavior by adopting the guidelines, with the intent of improving patient care, patient outcomes, and quality of life (McCormick 1988). Targeted groups such as consumers, health care practitioners, the health care industry, policymakers, researchers, and the media must be involved (Van Amringe & Shannon, 1992).

Guideline Defined

A guideline describes a process of patient care management that will facilitate improvement or maintenance of health status or slow the decline of health status in selected chronic clinical conditions. It has the potential for improving the quality of clinical and consumer decision-making. The guideline is *patient-centered,* rather than provider-centered.

The Office of the Forum (AHCPR) has published several clinical practice guidelines such as:

- *Acute Pain Management: Operative or Medical Procedures and Trauma*
- *Urinary Incontinence in Adults*
- *Pressure Ulcers in Adults: Prediction and Prevention*

Data Needed for Additional Guideline Development

- Identification of guidelines embedded in standards of practice, standardized care plans, protocols, core curricula, and statements of specialty organizations;
- A centralized database for existing guidelines;
- Identification of nursing variables that are common to many clinical conditions;
- A mechanism for capturing expert clinical knowledge necessary to develop clinical practice guidelines;
- Identification of clinical conditions characterized by high risks or potentially great benefits for individuals;
- Data for conditions for which wide variations exist among different treatment options and outcomes;
- Data for conditions in which current services and procedures are costly; and
- Data for conditions for which evaluation data are readily available or can be developed.

As guidelines are developed and implemented, nurse researchers should generate ideas and identify research questions. Guideline development provides an opportunity for nurse researchers to establish the scientific basis of nursing practice and to communicate that knowledge into outcome measures that can be quantified.

Criteria to Evaluate Health Policy Decisionmaking

What would one look for to measure the success of health policies being implemented?

- More even distribution of personal health services throughout the country, with an ample supply of health personnel and a variety of incentives available for improving access.
- Removal or lowering of major financial barriers to health services delivery for the most vulnerable groups—the poor, aged, and disabled.
- Demonstration by state and local governments and portions of the private sector of readiness to provide for personal health services.

- Establishment of a responsive health information system that is comprehensive and sensitive, so as to permit effective monitoring and corrections of health care actually provided.
- Improvement of organizational capabilities of state and local governments and the private sector.

If the present system of health care delivery is to be changed in a positive way, bold and provocative health policies (e.g., American Nurses Association 1992) are necessary.

Nursing Research and the Restructuring of the Nation's Health Care System

Nursing research can affect the coming changes in the health care system in many positive ways. Important changes to be addressed in nursing research include greater use of nurses as primary care providers, the effectiveness of emphasizing out-of-hospital care, and nurses' positions in new systems of care, such as managed care.

A survey conducted by the *American Journal of Nursing* (AJN) verified that nurses in general hospitals and nursing homes are performing—mostly without medical supervision—exactly the same services for which physicians are being reimbursed. These are based on CPT-coded services listed in the *Physicians' Current Procedural Terminology (CPT) Manual* published by the American Medical Association. Federal programs, such as Medicare and Medicaid, as well as private insurers use these codes when reimbursing physicians for these services (Griffith, Thomas & Griffith, 1991).

Examples of top ranked tasks performed by nurses for which physicians are reimbursed:

CPT-Coded Service	Percentage Performed by RNs
IM/SC Injection	95
Telephone Consultation	93
CPR	89
Urethral Catheterization	89
IV Injection	87
Suctioning	84
IM Antibiotic Injection	83
Starting IV	78
Bladder Irrigation	76
IV Infusion	76

Why are these data so significant? Physician payment reform to put a cap on escalating medical care costs would mean restructuring Medicare-Part B—a major source of physicians' payments. Nurse leaders for the most part ignored the impact of diagnosis-related groups (DRGs) on nursing by not insisting, from the first on inclusion of cost components for nursing services for each DRG. Lack of data about costs and outcome measures has made the nursing profession retroactive in its response rather than proactive.

Nowhere is it said that nurses providing physician services can be paid at lower rates to reduce costs. The databases needed to determine the basis for reimbursement of nursing care can be determined by nursing research. Information is needed about essential services, their impact on the patient/client, and where they can best be delivered. Such information must be readily available to health policymakers (Davis, 1988).

The Rand Study

The Rand Health Insurance Experiment uncovered inappropriate hospital admissions by physicians. Hospitalizing persons who could be treated on an outpatient basis or through a home care program adds significantly to health care costs (Siu, Manning, & Benjamin, 1990). There are a number of new ways to deal with high costs by such innovations as surgical care done on an outpatient basis.

Needed Restructuring of Hospitals

It is essential to reassess the role of hospitals. Today the technological base of modern medicine and the structure of health insurance payments make the hospital the dominant institution in the health care delivery system. Hospitals are expensive; physician reimbursement practices encourage specialization and reliance on expensive technology; and, finally, the hospital perpetuates the physician-centered medical model of cure rather than prevention. This results in the withholding of status and respect from other health professionals and in the loss of potential savings by denying the broader use of nonphysicians. Eighty percent of the hospital-based health care delivery services now provided by hospitals could be shifted to alternative facilities, e.g., HMOs or other ambulatory centers; birthing clinics; community mental health centers; home care programs; and self-help support groups.

What would be required?

- Changing the financial incentives to discourage overutilization of hospital-based services and limitation of the growth of specialization;
- Restraining hospitals from deterring the development of nonhospital and community-based services, for example, home care programs, birthing clinics, primary care health clinics, and self-support groups;
- Enlarging boards of trustees to include a majority of consumer representatives;
- Shifting the base of training and education to nonhospital settings (the teaching nursing home concept is an excellent shift in this direction);
- Enhancing the role of nonphysician health professionals (e.g., nurse practitioners and nurse midwives) within the hospital setting to afford them a key role in decisionmaking, hospital privileges, and access to patients;
- Encouraging hospital administrators and trustees to question the necessity of maintaining their hospital with its existing array of services; and
- Encouraging the development of economic incentives that will minimize regulation and place reliance on innovative approaches to other cost-containment methods that have proven to be effective.

Any proposal to manipulate incentives as a health policy device must be responsive to three questions: (1) Who must be made subject to the incentives if the desired outcome is to occur? (2) How do these individuals define rewards and penalties? (3) How large must the inducement be to bring about the desired outcome?

Managed Care

The concept of managed care is being looked on as a solution to the health care crisis. Managed care is health care provided by health maintenance organizations (HMOs) as well as companies that contract with hospitals and doctors to create looser networks of providers for members. (See Figure 11.4). Managed care companies closely scrutinize the type and frequency of procedures used in an effort to be more cost-efficient. HMOs and managed care networks do, and will in the future, make greater use of nonphysician providers such as nurse practitioners.

ELEMENTS OF 'MANAGED COMPETITION'

"managed competition. Under the broad outlines of the concept, most people would purchase health insurance from large, HMO-like managed-care networks that would compete for customers in a given region. A federally created board would set up nonprofit insurance purchasing organizations to bargain with networks for the most favorable rates.

INDIVIDUALS   SMALL BUSINESSES   LARGE BUSINESSES

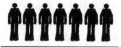 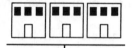 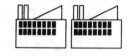

HEALTH PLAN PURCHASING COOPERATIVE

A government-established nonprofit agency (there could be one in each state or in each region of a state) acts as a price negotiator between the consumer who needs health benefits and qualified ("accountable") health plans who sell it.

ACCOUNTABLE HEALTH PLAN

The various approved health plans would probably be organized by insurers who create large networks of doctors, hospitals, clinics, and the like. It is likely that most of these would evolve into "super-HMOs," in which medical services and physician practices are scrutinized for cost-effectiveness and medical appropriateness.

AHPs cannot base rates on medical   All AHPs must at least offer
history or pre-existing conditions   the same basic benefits

NATIONAL HEALTH BOARD

Standardize accounting and paperwork; establish a standard benefits package

Provide consumer information on the quality of AHPs, including price and outcome information

Make a subsidy payment to plans with a large number of sick people so that no plan suffers disproportionately

Source: Rep. Jim Cooper (D–Tenn.)

Figure 11.4 Elements of managed competition.

Whatever national health plan is considered, nurses must insist on the following points:

1. Direct access to patients, with nurses as independent reimbursed practitioners;
2. Nurses to be the primary caregivers and nurse managers.

3. Nurses to sit on planning and regulatory commissions; and
4. Nursing services to be included in mandated benefits.

To play an active role in the development of a national health plan, nurses must be able to document what they do, and specify the costs and the benefits. Many health problems, such as drug and alcohol abuse, AIDS, teenage pregnancy, high infant mortality, and youth homicide, result from the widespread erosion of the family in our society. Nurses, as responsible health care professionals, must address the needs of the family at all levels of health care policy and involve the family in the solution of health problems.

This is an exciting time for nursing. The health system is in a great state of flux, and nurses can have significant impact on the system that emerges from this period of change. Nurse researchers can give policymakers a sound scientific basis for shaping more humane, less costly, and more inclusive health care for all (Pender, 1992b).

Chapter 12

The Funding of Nursing Research

N urse investigators must seek, find, and develop an awareness of the importance of receiving their share of available resources. Funds for nursing research and research training are mainly supplied by the federal government, nursing organizations, private foundations, universities, and industry. As federal funds dwindle and many individuals compete for the same funds, nonfederal funding in the form of seed grants and pilot studies becomes more significant. Nurse investigators must seek and find whatever sources are willing to invest in studies.

The Funding Crisis Affecting the New Investigator

The National Academy of Sciences' Institute of Medicine, troubled by the funding crisis affecting the new researcher, held a national forum in 1990 to highlight the issues and develop options toward their resolution (Institute of Medicine, 1990). Following is a discussion of the findings of the forum.

Dimensions of the Issue

Of the total U.S. outlay for health care in 1993, $800 billion, about 1.8%, was allocated for research, as compared to 2.6% by West Germany and 2.8% by Japan. The National Institutes of Health (NIH) budget is currently at an all-time high of $9.5 billion, but the number of new investigator invited awards (beginning grants known as RO1s) declined from 6,400 in 1988 to 4,600 in 1990. The chances of this type of grant being funded in 1970 was 50%; in 1990 it was 25%. These grants are vital to introducing young investigators to the research arena. Why does this funding crisis exist?

Contributing Factors

Well aware that few dollars are available for RO1 grants, established funded researchers demand that their grants be awarded for 4 to 5 years rather than 3 years, arguing that a longer time is necessary to investigate their topics.

Researchers submit multiple applications to improve their chances of getting funded. (The average researcher submits 1.9 grant applications.) Investigators with multiple applications do have a greater success rate, and multiple grants awarded to one researcher naturally reduce the chances of new investigators being funded (Fuller, Hasselmeyer, Hunter, Abdellah, & Hinshaw, 1991). Established researchers with a proven track record are more likely to be funded than new investigators, which defeats the purpose of RO1 Grants.

The NIH lacks a long-range strategy that would determine the criteria to be used to award quality grants and the proportion that should be new investigator awards.

The goals of current research should be scrutinized. Public policy thus far has directed health care providers to diagnose and treat illness. No savings from research will be forthcoming until public policy places a value on altering lifestyles, reduces its preoccupation with treatment, and focuses on prevention of disease and promotion of wellness.

Effects on the Researcher and the Research Institution

The increasing social importance and public awareness of new health technology make it essential that new researchers be recognized as the guardians of future scientific endeavors, otherwise they might become "endangered species." What are some of the effects on the new investigator who is unable to receive funding?

When new researchers fail to receive federal support in the first few years (with a 50% chance of approval and a 25% chance of funding), their careers as researchers often grind to a halt and they must seek other career routes. The future of scientific research, including nursing research, depends on an infusion of young, well-trained people with original ideas, fresh insights, and a willingness to trod new paths.

As research funds become more scarce, there is stress on the peer review system, as long-time researchers are well-known to their colleagues and new researchers not at all (White, 1991). The boundary between supporting or not supporting an outstanding proposal may be difficult to discern, and those with novel and interesting ideas may fall by the wayside.

Senior investigators worry about competing renewals and share their stress with graduate students, in some instances they may encourage them to abandon research as a career. Lack of funding can break up research teams.

Many predict a severe shortage of scientists and engineers by the year 2000. Although the American higher education system has not responded to this shift in goals, it has not produced enough graduates who are interested in and who qualify for these rigorous professions.

Setting Priorities for Research Funding

Priority setting must reflect the major professional and societal issues confronting the nursing discipline and must systematically order these according to their importance. (Block, 1990; Hinshaw, 1988a).

Criteria for Priority-Setting

- An area that represents a major current or future health care need;
- An area that is on the cutting edge of science, with the potential to contribute to new knowledge;
- An area constituting an opportunity for nursing to contribute to basic research, or a unique opportunity for nursing practice research with a readiness to identify outcomes measures; or

- An area that represents a costly health care burden for patients and/or the health care delivery system, offering a potential for cost savings.

Selected Federal Funding Sources That Give Priority to Health Policy Research

Agency for Health Care Policy and Research (AHCPR)

As discussed in the last chapter, pp. 204–205, the Agency for Health Care Policy and Research (AHCPR) was established in December 1989 as the successor to the National Center for Health Services Research and Health Care Technology assessment. The purpose of the Agency is to enhance the quality, appropriateness, and effectiveness of health care services through the establishment of a broad base of scientific research and promotion of improvements in clinical practice and in the organization, financing, and delivery of health care services.

Clinical Practice Guidelines and Quality Standards

AHCPR has a program to arrange for the development, periodic review, and updating of clinically relevant practice guidelines. These guidelines may be used by health care practitioners, educators, and consumers to help determine how various health conditions can most effectively be prevented, diagnosed, treated, and managed medically.

The program also develops quality assurance and medical review criteria that can be used by providers and other organizations to assess or review the quality and delivery of health care. These activities are carried out with the active involvement of health care providers, professional groups, and consumer organizations.

Other Extramural Research

AHCPR invites investigator-initiated research grants on such topics as:

- Assessment of health care technologies;
- Medical malpractice and liability;
- Delivery of health services in rural areas;

- Availability, accessibility, and quality of care for low-income groups, minorities, and the elderly; and
- Alternative delivery systems, providers, and practice patterns with HIV-related illnesses.

Database Development

AHCPR supports the design and development of new databases and enhancement of existing databases for use in patient outcomes research and clinical decisionmaking. Areas of support include the development of uniform definitions for patient data, common reporting formats, database linkages, and security and confidentiality standards. AHCPR supports investigations of the uniformity and relevance of data for medical effectiveness research; the representation of minority populations in databases; and the promotion of wide access to these data.

In cooperation with AHCPR, the National Library of Medicine will review and enhance the treatment of health services research information and literature in all its basic services and look at new ways to disseminate the results of health services research to health professions and the public.

Information Dissemination and Liaison

AHCPR is expanding its information dissemination activities in order to make health services research information available and useful to a wide range of decisionmakers. The Agency will support demonstrations of improved methods for disseminating research findings.

The Office of the Forum for Quality and Effectiveness in Health Care is responsible for developing and updating guidelines to be used in the management of clinical conditions. These guidelines are formulated as part of the Medical Treatment Effectiveness Program, which also includes database development, effectiveness and outcomes research, and dissemination of research findings and guidelines.

Algorithm Approach to Clinical Guideline Development

A useful publication using an algorithm approach to clinical guideline development discusses two algorithms from the Urinary Incontinence in Adults Guideline Panel, employing systematic annotation to link the algorithms' recommendations to the literature, and patient counseling and decision nodes to show major preference-dependent branch points in the algorithm (Urinary Incontinence Guideline Panel, 1992).

As guidelines are developed and reviewed, nurse researchers should generate ideas and identify research questions to encourage further development, and communicate them to appropriate professional and research organizations such as the National Institute of Nursing Research. Guidelines must be based upon available scientific knowledge and expert consensus and begin in those areas for which there is currently established research and a high degree of consensus.

For additional information, write to: Agency for Health Care Policy and Research, Executive Office Center, Suite 300, 2101 East Jefferson Street, Rockville, MD 20852. Phone: (301) 227–6662.

National Institute of Nursing Research

Seven priorities were approved for development by the National Advisory Council for Nursing Research at its June 1988 meeting. Cross-cutting issues are inherent in all priority areas.

The seven priorities are (Block, 1990):

Stage I:

Low birth weight: Mothers and infants.   This priority includes study of the nursing care of prospective mothers at risk for having a low-birthweight infant, with a focus on prevention of premature delivery; and of the care of low-birthweight infants, with a focus on prevention of complications.

HIV infection: Prevention and care.   Prevention, ethical issues, and physiological/psychosocial factors relating to care of persons with AIDS or HIV infection need to be examined.

Stage II:

Long-term care for the elderly.   Possible areas to be developed include quality of nursing care, continuity of care, and iatrogenic complications. Important issues related to self-care, patient and caregiver coping and adaptation, and care of special populations such as the frail elderly need to be addressed.

Symptom management.   The priority should blend biopsychosocial parameters of patient symptoms, such as pain, fatigue, nausea and vomiting, and include acute, chronic, and terminal care. Measures for symptom assessment and management need to be developed.

Information systems. Standardized datasets that document nursing care across settings and a taxonomy to classify nursing phenomena and allow for the common use of terms are needed. The link(s) between resources and patient outcomes needs to be developed.

Stage III:

Health promotion. The critical issue for study is the psychosocial mechanism underlying health promotion behaviors, with emphasis on lifestyle and the need to take responsibility for one's own health. Special population groups, such as children and the handicapped, need to be targeted.

Technology dependency across the lifespan. The interest here is in technology dependency, individual and family responses to technology, and prevention of iatrogenic complications from the use of technology.

Additional New Initiatives Include:

- *Research for understanding the dysfunctioning bladder and bowel.* Diagnostic procedures and developments in functional neuromuscular stimulation are among the advances offering opportunities for researchers to improve techniques.
- *Nursing and biology interface.* There is a critical need to explore innovative, state-of-the-art biological techniques to solve nursing problems and clinical questions.
- *Home health care and supportive services for older adults.* Research is encouraged on in-home care for older, dependent Americans.
- *Interventions to manage Alzheimer's disease symptoms.* Nursing research can make a significant contribution to improving the care and management of Alzheimer's patients.
- *Community-based care for chronically ill older Americans.* Research is needed to find ways to delay institutionalization.
- *Long-term care and minority aging.* Research is needed on long-term care of minorities who tend not to use formal care arrangements as they age.

- *Biobehavioral symptom management.* Much needed is research of innovative clinical assessment and management of symptoms.
- *Minority youth health behavior research.* Research is needed of the development and evaluation of interventions (National Center for Nursing Research, 1992).

NINR's Agenda for the Year 2000

A second Conference on Research Priorities was held in November 1992 to recommend an updated set of research priorities to form the National Nursing Research Agenda for the year 2000 (National Center for Nursing Research, 1992d). This research agenda is intended to promote depth in nursing science vital to the health of the American people.

Priority statements resulting from the 1992 conference include:

- *Community-based Nursing Models* (1995)
  Develop and test community-based nursing models designed to promote access to, utilization of, and quality of health services by rural and other underserved populations.

- *Effectiveness of Nursing Interventions in HIV/AIDS* (1996)
  Assess the effectiveness of biobehavioral nursing interventions to foster health-promoting behaviors of individuals at risk for HIV/AIDS, and of biobehavioral interventions to ameliorate the effects of illness in individuals who are already infected. The focus is on individuals of different cultural backgrounds—especially women. The need to incorporate biobehavioral markers is noted.

- *Cognitive Impairment* (1997)
  Develop and test biobehavioral and environmental approaches to remediating cognitive impairment.

- *Living with Chronic Illness* (1998)
  Test interventions to strengthen individuals' personal resources in dealing with chronic illness.

- *Biobehavioral Factors Related to Immunocompetence* (1999)
  Identify biobehavioral factors and test interventions to promote immunocompetence.

Plans are to implement one priority a year, after refinement of each priority area by a newly constituted multidisciplinary Priority Expert Panel (PEP), (National Institute of Nursing Research, 1993).

For additional information, reference should be made to NINR staff.

Questions that need to be raised about funding by NINR:

- *How do I decide when to apply for a research grant and which one to apply for?*
  The choice of support mechanism depends on the investigator's needs and skills. The NINR Division of Extramural Programs can provide consultation. For additional information and applications write to the National Institute of Nursing Research, National Institutes of Health, 9000 Rockville Pike, Bethesda, MD 20892.

- *How do I obtain application forms?*
  If not available at your institution, write to: NIH Division of Research Grants, Room 449, Westwood Building, Bethesda, MD 20892. Request the NIH Publication (1993) *Preparing a Research Grant Application to the National Institutes of Health.*

- *How are applications for research grants reviewed?*
  Figure 12.1 shows the grant review process. Proposals are reviewed in three grant cycles. Final date for submission and minimum time to allow is 10 months. Dates for new research grants are February 1, June 1, and October 1; for competing continuation, supplemental and revised grants the dates are March 1, July 1, and November 1.

A study of approved applications by NINR documented that approved applications addressed meaningful problems of sufficient size and of importance to warrant study; had a well-synthesized literature review; and were solvable by available techniques. In addition, research plans were consonant with the aims of the research, and the methods sections reflected the investigator's understanding of the principles underlying the techniques. Also existing were a supportive environment and adequate research resources, including access to study populations. On the other hand, disapproved applications had a poor synthesis of the literature; methods were inconsistent with aims; and the investigator showed a lack of understanding of the techniques (Fuller, Hasselmeyer, Hunter, Abdellah, & Hinshaw, 1991).

Division of Nursing, Bureau of Health Professions, Health Resources and Services Administration, U.S. Public Health Service

The Division of Nursing (DN) is the key federal focus for nursing education and practice. It provides national leadership to assure an

NIH Research Grant Application Review Process

National Institutes of Health (NIH)

Investigator
Initiates research idea
Develops application

Research Institution or School
Submits application to
NIH Division of Research Grants (DRG)

NIH Division of Research Grants (DRG)
Assigns applications relevant to nursing
research to appropriate initial review group and
to appropriate NIH funding unit (usually NCNR)

Initial Review Group
Evaluates for scientific merit
Recommends approval, disapproval, or deferral
Assigns priority score to approved applications

NIH Funding Unit
Evaluates for program relevance

National Advisory Council for Funding Unit
Recommends action

Director of Funding Unit
Takes final action for NIH Director

Research Institution or School
Receives and manages funds

Investigator
Conducts research

Source: National Center for Nursing Research (1992a) *Facts About funding* (NIH Publication No. 92–3112). Bethesda, MD: National Institutes of Health.

Figure 12.1 Overview of the grant-review process.

adequate supply and distribution of qualified nursing personnel to meet the health needs of the nation (Table 12.1, Funding for DN and NINR).

Division of Nursing strategic directions:

- Enhancing nursing's contributions to primary health care and public health;

TABLE 12.1

Nursing Education and Research Funding ($ in millions)

	FY93	FY92
Advanced Education	12.2	12.3
Nurse Practioner/CNM	15.4	14.5
Special Projects	10.9	10.4
Traineeships	14.1	13.9
Nurse Anesthetist	1.9	2.7
Disadvantaged Assistance	3.3	3.6
Undergraduate Scholarships	0	2.3
Loan Repayment	1.4	2.0
Total Education	59.2	61.7
Nursing Research	48.2	44.9

The American Nurse, November–December 1992

- Developing and promoting innovative practice models for improved and expanded nursing services;
- Enhancing racial and ethnic diversity and cultural competency in the nursing workforce;
- Promoting improved and expanded linkages between education and practice;
- Improving and expanding nursing services to high-risk and underserved populations;
- Enhancing nursing's contributions to achieving the *Healthy People 2000* objectives and health care reform; and
- Capacity building for meeting the nursing service needs of the nation.

For additional information and applications write to the Division of Nursing, Bureau of Health Professions, Room 9-35, Parklawn Building, 5600 Fishers Lane, Rockville, MD 20857. Phone: (301) 443–6333.

Federal Office of Rural Health Policy

The Office of Rural Health Policy (ORHP) was established within the Health Resources and Services Administration (DHHS/PHS) in 1987. The major responsibility of this office is to work within the Department and with other federal agencies, states, national associations, foundations, and private sector organizations to seek solutions to health care problems in rural communities.

Rural Health Outreach Grant Program

This program supports projects that demonstrate new and innovative models of health care delivery in rural areas to improve the integration and coordination of rural health services. Grants are awarded to consortia of three or more existing health care or social service providers. Nonprofit rural hospitals, clinics, medical/nurse group practices, public health agencies, and community health centers are eligible for grants as part of these consortia. Profitmaking organizations may be part of a consortium.

Rural Health Research

A Rural Health Research Center grant program was initiated in 1988. These centers collect and analyze information, conduct applied research on rural health issues, and widely disseminate the results. Current centers participating in the program are the Universities of Washington, North Dakota, Minnesota, Southern Maine, North Carolina, Florida and at the University of New York at Buffalo. The University of Nebraska's Rural Health Center is completing a series of policy briefs analyzing the rural consequences of various health care reform proposals.

For further information and assistance contact: Public Affairs Director, Office of Rural Health Policy, 5600 Fishers Lane, Room 9–05, Rockville, MD 20857. Phone: (301) 443-0835. FAX: (301) 443-2803.

The National Library of Medicine Extramural Grants Programs

The National Library of Medicine's (NLM) extramural research programs provide grants for research and development activities leading to the better management, dissemination, and use of medical/nursing knowledge. Improved biomedical communication and knowledge access are essential if the nation is to exploit the findings of health research in the advancement of medical and nursing education, practice, and research.

Research Grant Program

Grant support is available for a variety of scientific investigations and activities regarding health knowledge issues. Projects supported can range from highly theoretical studies to development applications. There are three program areas:

- *Medical/nursing informatics.* This area includes studies of health knowledge representation, retrieval, and utilization in the context of advanced computer technology. An example would be work on an intelligent expert system for managing cancer therapy protocols.
- *Health information science.* This area includes studies of bibliographic organization and retrieval of recorded biomedical knowledge. An example would be an evaluation of alternate retrieval capabilities for computerized medical/nursing bibliographies.
- *Biotechnology information.* This area includes investigations of more effective methodologies for organizing and analyzing vast amounts of data and information relating to molecular control of life processes. An example would be a general pattern matching algorithm for biological sequences.

Training and Fellowships

NLM supports research training in the fields of medical/nursing informatics and biotechnology information. The general purpose is to prepare individuals to address fundamental issues which will advance the frontiers of the computer sciences for organizing, retrieving, and utilizing health knowledge.

Publication Grant Program

Grants are available to provide financial assistance for the preparation and publication of important scientific publications needed by health professionals and which are not commercially viable. Supported studies include critical reviews and monographs on current and past developments in medical/nursing research and services, publications in health sciences, and biomedical communications and handbooks.

Resource Grants

The purpose of this type of grant is to improve information services to health science professionals.

Information Access Grants for Health Science Libraries

These grants are intended for libraries of small to medium-size community hospitals and to consortia of health-related libraries to facilitate access to and delivery of health science information, employing the most up-to-date and effective computer and telecommunications technology available.

Information Systems Grants for Health Science Institutions

These grants are given to health science academic institutions and to hospitals with significant teaching and research components. Their purpose is to utilize and improve the infrastructure for the transfer of health science information via technological means.

IAIMS Program

Integrated Academic Information Management Systems (IAIMS) use computer and communications networks to transform a health institution's various information bases into an integrated system. The goal is to link and relate the databases representing academic information. For example, the published knowledge base and bibliographic records are integrated into individual and institutional working information files, such as clinical, administrative, research, and education data bases.

   For additional information and assistance contact: The National Library of Medicine, Extramural Programs, 8600 Rockville Pike, Bethesda, MD 20894. Phone: (301) 496–4621.

Health Fundraising in the Private Sector

For information on health fundraising in the private sector, see *The National Guide to Funding in Health* (2nd Ed.), published by The Foundation Center, 79 Fifth Avenue/16th Street, New York, NY 10003–3037. Phone: (212) 620–4230 or (800) 424–9836. FAX: (212) 807–3677. This volume provides essential facts on more than 2,500 foundations and corporate direct giving programs.

Fellowships for Health Policy Research

The Agency for Health Care Policy and Research supports postdoctoral fellowships in health services research through the National Research Service Award program. These fellowships are intended to address the nation's current and future needs for health services researchers. Opportunity is provided for full-time training in methods of analyzing and evaluating issues and problems related to the organization, financing, delivery, and utilization of health services.

Application must be made on Form PHS 416-1 and submitted to the Division of Research Grants, National Institutes of Health. Fellowship applications are available from the Director, Office of Scientific Review, AHCPR, Executive Office Center, 2101 East Jefferson Street, Suite 602, Rockville, MD 20852. Phone: (301) 277–8449.

Funding Strategy

Improving outcomes and quality of care are identified by agencies supporting health policy research as high priority areas. Without inclusion of data for nursing, the validity of the data system is compromised (Hinshaw, 1988b; National Center for Nursing Research, 1989).

In view of escalating costs and generally diminishing funds in the health care system in the United States, nursing research, as part of the system with the largest number of members who spend the largest amount of health care time, has much to contribute to the future viability of the system by its contributions to basic knowledge and methodology.

Options for Action

Nurse researchers need to make a greater effort to let society know about the benefits of nursing research. This means translating research findings into practice that both the nurse practitioner and patient/client can understand and see as a benefit.

Improvement in the "quality of life" does result from research. Nurse researchers must see that the public/patient knows and understands that what they have done is new and better and will benefit them. It will take a concerted effort to communicate nursing research findings to consumers, the media, and health policy decisionmakers.

Administrators, deans, and department chairs must be encouraged to give recognition to the needs of new researchers. The new nurse researcher should be counselled and helped to obtain initial funding from such sources as Sigma Theta Tau, the American Nurses' Foundation, industry, and private philanthropy. After 1 to 3 years of successful experience, the researcher should be encouraged to apply for investigator awards from federal sources. Originality, creativity, insightful perception, and even unconventional vision are the lifeblood of a dynamic and vibrant science; these questions must be recognized and encouraged, and not allowed to wither away.

The establishing of different priorities for RO1 awards should be considered for the use of existing monies while focusing on quality. Quality may suffer when grants are awarded within a targeted program or by mechanisms outside the RO1 type award, due to fewer controls.

A positive research environment for health sciences can be created by identifying and encouraging talented individuals to pursue health research careers; providing stable research support for talented researchers throughout their careers; providing flexibility in allocating resources; and providing modern laboratories and equipment essential for scientific research and training.

Partnerships with industries need to be encouraged to support and invest in new nurse researchers and to commit 10% of their R & D budget to them. The quality of nursing research must be upgraded. The scientist and practitioner can enhance the quality of research by a closer partnership and collaboration.

The most critical and long-term investment is the development of career scientists who can contribute to the long-term success of the research and the training of future scientists.

To achieve long-term goals in health science research requires a priority setting framework; reallocation of resources to achieve an appropriate balance among people, projects, facilities, and equipment; and the establishment of communication channels between sponsors and researchers. Especially needed are programs to be developed by the federal government, the private sector, and the education sector that are designed to encourage and enable more women and minorities to pursue careers in health science and health policy research.

To achieve a more active role in health policy research and in the policy decision process, investigators need to serve on peer review panels, review journal articles, and provide advice on health policy to health policymakers. The responsibility of the scientist to communicate research findings to the public should be seen as one more facet of the entire spectrum of responsibilities encompassed in the research domain (Bloom & Randolph, 1990). Much attention needs to be paid as to how best to deliver research findings rapidly.

The federal government needs to conduct long-range planning across the sciences, both for research and training needs. What is accomplished in planning in this decade governs the actuality of the future. Nurses need to have input into the health policy planning process. The level of funds for new researchers needs to be specified in balance with funds for senior investigators and research training.

Much needed in nursing is a constituency for science and research to communicate the benefits of nursing research to Congress and the public. Nurses should pay particular attention to those people in Congress who are interested and can relate nursing research findings to their legislative programs. As more women become active in politics at all levels of government, but especially as members of Congress, prospects brighten that women's issues, including health issues, will be given the more serious attention and action that they deserve. Nurse researchers need to take responsibility for their own destiny! One way in which this can be accomplished is through participation in such organizations as Research! America, a coalition of universities, industry, and philanthropy with one mission, namely to educate the Congress and the public about research. This group forms a powerful alliance for discoveries in health. Nursing can benefit by becoming more actively involved in such an alliance.

For additional information about Research! America write to: Suite 250, 99 Canal Center Plaza, Alexandria, VA 22314. Phone: (703) 739–2577; FAX: (703) 739–2372.

Chapter 13

Future Challenges

To develop a realistic agenda for research priorities for the year 2000, it is important to identify the current gaps in nursing research. This chapter will identify these gaps and identify priority areas for future research and strategic planning.

Current Gaps in Nursing Research

After almost four decades of federal government support of nursing research, what gaps still exist?

Clinical Research

Clinical research of problems related to nursing practice is considered a high priority. There is a dearth of descriptive data about physiological and behavioral phenomena of patients with varied diagnoses and in varied settings.

Advances in clinical research in nursing require the following: precise measuring instruments, identification of criterion measures of quality nursing practice, and development of models and theories that have relevance for nursing. In addition to lacks in these areas, nurse investigators do not have ready access to study populations or to animal laboratories. Until these obstacles are overcome, the scientific basis of nursing practices cannot be studied in depth.

Some measure of progress has been achieved in areas of parent and child health, care of the premature infant, and care of the aged. But the health needs of the majority of individuals with multiple health problems who fall within the center of the health needs/health care spectrum have remained largely unexplored. Little is known about the dynamics of patient care systems; for example, how patients cope with their health problems; how risky health behaviors are changed; and how the costs of nursing services provided are determined.

Finally, nursing presently makes only limited use of instrumental monitoring devices to assist in analyses of patient care data important to predicting outcomes.

Theory Development

The lack of tested nursing theories is a major gap. More knowledge is needed on sources of nursing theory, the components of theories, and the development of theories.

Few studies have specifically focused on model and theory development. The scientific basis for nursing interventions for all nursing diagnoses needs to be identified. Nursing practice criteria need to be defined explicitly for all problems.

Measurement of Patient Care Systems

The precise measurement of patient care provided depends upon the development of standards (clinical practice guidelines). These standards can be derived from actual nursing practice or from expert judgment. Nursing is beginning to define the prerequisites for nursing care for groups of patients with common nursing diagnoses and problems among different age groups, and in different settings. Educational aspects of health promotion and disease prevention become significant.

The evaluation of nursing performance takes on new importance. Here such observable quantitative measures can be used as the time nursing personnel spend on activities with patients; utilization rates for specific procedures; and length of patient stay in relation to intensity of nursing services.

Criterion measures of patient care and precise instrumentation to measure the effects of nursing practice upon patient care are major gaps in nursing research. The complex nature of studying patient care systems is clearly evident by the gaps in this area. There has been some progress in looking at organizational patterns of health services, but these have been predominantly hospital-based.

There are also major gaps in methods of research that are applicable to the study of patient care systems. The methodological gap includes the need for greater accuracy and control of instruments, interview schedules, and observational methods. Medical and nursing records need to be computerized to provide more useful and comparative data. Needed are research tools to measure the effectiveness (both objective and subjective) of health services provided; indices of total performance; improved nursing research designs; and criteria of quality nursing care.

Role Behaviors

Most of the studies on role behaviors of nurses have used behavioral science techniques, with only limited involvement of nurses in the research process. There is a paucity of research in nursing that directly measures the extent to which medical and surgical nursing personnel actually differ in their performance and the effect of their practice on patients. What and where are the differences in the approach to the patient of the two groups, and how is the patient affected, if at all? Lacking are descriptive studies of nurse behaviors, nurse-patient behaviors, and nurse-physician behaviors.

Nursing Students

Further research is needed about intellectual, personal, and other characteristics that distinguish successful from unsuccessful students. Reliable tests are needed to predict clinical performance. Lacking is research that has examined occupational choice longitudinally.

Some progress has been made in developing methods for selecting and preparing nursing students, with greater emphasis on meeting the individual needs of students by offering multiple bridges to achieving career goals.

Policy Decisionmaking and Liability Protection for Health Care Providers

Attention must be given to liability protection for health care providers. The number of lawsuits against nurses has increased considerably in recent years. The average award in a claim against a nurse is $39,200. A sound program of personal risk management and a plan of professional liability insurance can help to avoid costly malpractice suits. As lawsuits increase, nurses are named in many of the actions. Insurance industry experts predict that the nation could be facing a major liability insurance crisis (*Averting Liability Crisis is the Goal*, 1991).

Malpractice tort. The Agency for Health Care Policy and Research (AHCPR) held a working conference from February 27 to March 1, 1991, to identify issues in medical liability. Health care decisionmaking, often affected by nonmedical factors in an effort to avoid adverse outcomes, can result in overutilization of diagnostic and treatment resources—i.e., defensive medicine. Other factors are: limitations on patient access to care that limits prevention and early treatment; increased liability insurance premiums; the effect of lawsuits on treatment decisions; medical care costs; education; and manpower.

Needed are efficient and cost-effective systems that will reduce health professional and facility errors; elimination of ineffective and obsolete treatments; additional development of practice guidelines; provider education; improved access to care; and measurement and monitoring of quality of delivered care.

Research needed includes:

- Demonstration projects on the effectiveness of sanctions and interventions;
- Study of causes of good or poor health care provider performance;
- Demonstration projects on payment effects—linkage to quality, patient satisfaction, and outcomes; and
- Study of malpractice premiums related to practitioner behavior.

Other Needs in Nursing Research:

- Study of the environment and how it impacts on health promotion and disease prevention;
- Historical research of nursing (25 years has elapsed since the works of noted nurse historians Mary Roberts and Teresa Christy were produced);
- Health economics—particularly costing out the nursing components of nursing practices;
- Medical, legal, and ethical aspects of nursing practices; and
- Health policy issues and how nurse researchers can use their research data to influence health policymakers.

Strategic Plan for Nursing Research

A strategic plan is essential in order to make sure that priority areas are identified, an implementation plan is thought through, and the budget needs specified.

To address the gaps in nursing research in the future, the following strategic plan is suggested:

Clinical research. As the 21st century approaches, major breakthroughs are bound to come from research in the biological and behavioral sciences that will result in the improvement of nursing practices. Nursing practices will undergo many changes as researchers successfully achieve tissue and organ transplants and the regeneration of tissues. A productive area of research will be the collection of descriptive data of patient behaviors as patients/clients react to and interact with physiological and environmental phenomena. Evaluation of patient care should be based upon systematic observations and studies of nurse actions and strategies that establish the scientific bases for nursing practice. Examples of studies include:

- The physiological and psychological behaviors of patients with different types of diagnoses in different environments that can predict the consequences of nursing interventions;
- Problems related to operation of patient monitoring devices, medical and treatment consoles;
- Inter- and intra-professional communication and the effects upon professional nursing practice;
- The diagnostic process: initiation, professional actions affecting it, patient involvement, and assessment of the patient's problems; and
- Utilization of every means possible to communicate scientific findings to nurses and to health policymakers so that they can be incorporated into practice.

Theory Development

Nursing theories result from the integration of nursing with the basic sciences and are drawn from the world of empirical reality. Knowledge is needed about behavior of patients with different diagnoses and of different demographic and economic backgrounds. Knowledge is also needed about patterns, processes, and phenomena in patient care situations.

Relevant theories need to be identified that would be useful in building the scientific bases of nursing practice. Once identified, these theories should be tested and validated.

Measurement of Patient Care Systems

Criterion measures of nursing practice must derive from outcome measures that indicate the effects of practice upon patient care. Criterion measures of patient care fall into four main groups:

Group I.   Criterion measures of patient care related to preventive care needs;

Group II.   Criterion measures of patient care related to normal and disturbed physiological body processes that are vital to sustaining life;

Group III.   Criterion measures of patient care related to rehabilitative needs; and

Group IV.   Criterion measures related to sociological and community problems affecting patient care.

Professional Practice Models

A major part of the future research effort needs to make full utilization of existing scientific knowledge and technologies in achieving effective organizational patterns of patient care systems.

Studies are needed of problems covering the supply and distribution of nursing resources and the logistics for managing them. Also needed are studies of the incidence of illness and accidents and the intensity and duration of the need for hospitalization.

Instrumentation, including the use of computers, promises fruitful changes in the organization and delivery of nursing services. Studies are needed of the dynamics of nursing recruitment, educational processes, and career patterns—and of the cultural, social, and psychological variables that influence these processes. These include comparative studies of competing occupational careers, factors affecting the demand and supply of nursing, job turnover, job satisfaction, and problems of adaptation of the nursing profession to technological, social, and cultural changes (Abdellah, 1970).

Violence and Public Health

More than 4 million victims of violence—from child abuse to elder abuse—cry out for help each year (U. S. Department of Health and Human Services, 1986). Former Surgeon General C. Everett Koop declared violence as the number one public health problem. Throughout history, the two leading causes of premature death have been infectious diseases and violence. Infectious disease control started 197 years ago with the work of Jenner, when he developed the first vaccine for smallpox. The solution of the problems of violence, on the other hand, has defied the best minds in health, politics, religion, and law enforcement. Violence must be recognized as a major public health problem that can no longer be ignored.

Research should be focused on the more vulnerable, high-risk populations—children, the elderly, and minorities. There is a need to determine the relationship between violence, the abuse of drugs and alcohol, and the family and its economic circumstances. Field models of effective intervention need to be developed. The relationship between abuse in childhood and high risk in adulthood needs to be determined. The investigation of privacy laws and law enforcement procedures need to be studied to learn what restrictions inhibit public health practices (U.S. Department of Health and Human Services, 1986).

NIH's Strategic Plan and How Nursing Fits Into the Plan

The National Institutes of Health (NIH) is the principal research arm of the U.S. Public Health Service, DHHS. NIH is the nation's and the world's largest sponsor of biomedical research. It has provided sustained support for basic and clinical biomedical investigations. The National Institute of Nursing Research (NINR) has been a part of NIH since 1986; called the Center for Nursing Research prior to 1993.

NIH's strategic plan builds on past accomplishments, organizational strengths, and mechanisms of proven value. The biomedical and behavioral sciences have entered an era of unprecedented opportunity—a new age of discovery and application. The NIH mission statement for the 21st century is focused science in pursuit of knowledge with the goal to extend healthy life and reduce the burdens of illness and disability (National Institutes of Health, 1992).

Following are five objectives by NIH in this statement for the 21st century:

Objective 1: Critical Science and Technology

Assure that critical science and technology in basic biology impacting on human health and the national economy are advanced as priorities across the NIH. Operational components include molecular medicine, biotechnology, molecular immunology and vaccine development, and structural biology.

Objective 2: Research Capacity

The capacity of the national biomedical and behavioral research enterprise to respond to current and emerging public health needs should be stregthened. Some operational components include basic biology and the environment, neuroscience and behavior, childhood health and mortality, reproductive biology and development, and prevention, health education, and disease control. Other needs to be addressed are: population-based studies, chronic and recurrent illnesses, aging, and the health of women, minorities, and underserved populations.

These objectives are treated in the DHHS/PHS's strategic plan, *Healthy People 2000* (U.S. Department of Health and Human Services, 1991).

Objective 3: Intellectual Capital

There is a need to provide for the renewal and growth of the intellectual capital base essential to the biomedical research enterprise. This can be done by ensuring fairness and equality of opportunity at NIH to enhance the human resource base of biomedical research. These operational components include science education and human resource development, intramural research, i.e., maintaining a research infrastructure, and attention to professional standards of scientific research.

Objective 4: The Stewardship of Public Resources

This requires that the scientific community secure the maximal return on the public investment in the enterprise. These operational components include technology transfer, cost management, and intramural research (research infrastructure).

Objective 5: Public Trust

The scientific community must continually earn the public's respect, trust, and confidence. This means giving attention to the social, legal, and ethical issues in biomedical and behavioral research, and adhering to professional standards of scientific research. Further, concern with science education and human resource development, communications and information flow, and the impact of research on the nation's economy, i.e., health care and biotechnology. Technology transfer must be demonstrated to be in the public interest. Scientists must be seen to care about the larger world outside science.

Pender (1992b) emphasizes the importance of reviewing NIH's strategic plan for its research implications for nursing. Will the areas targeted result in important breakthroughs in health care? Will critical technologies identified warrant major investment of NIH's resources? How can NIH and NINR join forces in recruiting promising students to careers in science? It has been noted that interest in research careers is decreasing.

Expansion of the Federal Government's Role in Defining Quality

Quality is related to productivity and accountability and must be part of the strategic plan. It is helpful to review historically how quality emerged, and how studies related to quality provided the basis for outcomes research almost three decades later.

Expansion of the federal government in health care began after World War II with the increased funding of biomedical research and hospital building as a result of the Hill-Burton Act, Medicare, Medicaid, and Title V programs. There was much interest in the application of new technologies that policymakers believed accelerated the high cost of care. In 1974, the federal government launched its quality assurance initiative, the Professional Standards Review Organization (PSRO), in an effort to contain costs. PSROs are organizations of locally practicing physicians who are given government grants to ensure that services provided to beneficiaries in federal programs are essential.

The federal government viewed quality as a desirable attribute, the worth of which must be weighed against cost. Donabedian defines quality of care as a judgment about the goodness of both technical care and the management of the interpersonal exchanges between client and practitioner (Palmer, Donabedian, & Povar, 1991). The quality of technical care is judged by its effectiveness, based on currently achievable improvements in health that the patient/client can be expected to attain. The emphasis on a more precise definition of quality laid the groundwork for the expansion of outcomes research.

Productivity and Health Care

Productivity is related to the current health care crisis. Health policy-makers, frustrated in their efforts to control costs, have introduced policies that change incentives for hospitals. Nurse researchers must become involved in assessing productivity. The concept of productivity has been a familiar concept in industry for decades. In nursing, the concept of productivity encompasses both the effectiveness of nursing care, which relates to quality and appropriateness, and the efficiency of care, which is production of nursing output with minimal resource waste (Jelinek & Dennis, 1976).

Quality of care is an essential component of productivity, and nurse researchers need to incorporate quality of care into definitions of productivity (Hegyvary, 1986). Curtin (1986) emphasized the importance of care provided to the patient and the patient be served successfully.

A seminal study conducted by Myrtle Aydelotte in 1973 reviewed research on staffing methodologies and identified specific areas for future research. The areas of needed research that she identified are still relevant today and provide a framework for the nurse researcher in projecting needed research in preparing for the 21st century. These areas are:

- Development of conceptual models of the nursing care delivery system;
- Defined studies of patient classification systems;
- Patient classification systems built around nurses' perceptions of care, nursing problems, nursing priorities, knowledge, and skill levels;
- Studies of the effect of improved support systems, e.g., patient care items, equipment, and supplies;
- A concentrated effort on the measurement of quality of care; and
- Guidelines for simultaneous use of different methodologies.

Efforts to define and measure nursing productivity have taken a great leap forward with the recognition of the importance of outcome measures and clinical practice guidelines. Needed is a system for monitoring nursing productivity. Additional efforts needed are:

- Further conceptual development of the nursing profession—its goals, purposes, knowledge base, activities, and its relationships with other providers;
- Improved tools to measure and monitor provider inputs;
- Improved measures of patient inputs, particularly patient classification based on needs for nursing care;
- Quantification of the quality of nursing performance;
- Quantification of patient outcomes; and
- Integration of all parts of the system—both measurement and management (Hegyvary, 1986).

Changing Functions and Responsibilities of Nurse Practitioners As Related to Nurse Productivity

The decade of the eighties brought about a proliferation of nurse practitioners who are managing care for less acute emergency patients in subacute or walk-in areas. So important has the nurse practitioner become to the delivery of primary health services in that all health care reform projections predict enormous shortages by the year 2000.

Nurse practitioners are not a new phenomenon. Henry Silver and Loretta Ford developed the first nurse practitioner programs in Colorado (Mallison, 1993). The acute shortage of primary care physicians has changed the situation, giving support for the nurse practitioner who handles admissions, manages daily treatments, and arranges for discharge. A study conducted by the American Nurses Association (ANA) found that nurse practitioners perform as well as or better than physicians in delivering primary health care (Brown & Grimes, 1993). Using meta-analysis to assess the effectiveness of nurse practitioner care when compared to physician care, the researchers included more than 38 studies of nurse practitioners (NPs) and 15 studies of certified nurse-midwives (CNMs).

Key findings of the ANA study documented that when compared to physicians:

- NPs provided more health promotion activities;
- NPs scored higher on quality of care measures;
- NPs achieved equivalent clinical outcomes or scored more favorably;

- Patients expressed greater satisfaction with care;
- NPs spent more time with patients on compliance with health promotion and treatment, recommendations, and health status; and
- The average cost per patient visit for NPs was significantly lower (39%).

Thus, nurse practitioners can provide more affordable care (primary care) at a high level of quality of care (Brown & Grimes, 1993). There is a trend to merge the nurse practitioner (NP) and clinical nurse specialist (CNS) into one advanced nurse practice provider. The National Institute of Nursing Research currently is supporting innovative practice models to stimulate studies that include demonstration and evaluation of community-based practice models targeted to minority populations. Three models are being implemented in Arizona, New York, and Baltimore.

The role of the nurse has changed dramatically. As members of the nursing profession move out of general staff nurse roles in hospitals, having gained new education and assuming new responsibilities in the developing and management of care, particularly in primary case settings, they are functioning in roles that are accountable to society (O'Neil, 1993).

Utilizing Advanced Technology: New Tools for the 21st Century

As we explore ways to improve health care delivery, we need to be aware of new tools for health policy research. Genetic research offers such a tool. Most genetic diseases are rare, but collectively constitute 3,000 known inherited disorders resulting from single altered genes that deprive millions of healthy and productive lives. The goal of NIH's Human Genome Project is to provide scientists with powerful new tools to clear research hurdles related to such devastating diseases as cancer, schizophrenia, alcoholism, Alzheimer's, Parkinson's, diabetes, and immune systems disorders, to name just a few. The development of new research tools by biomedical scientists requires attention to ethical, legal, and social health policy issues related to the use of these tools.

Computers in Research

The trend is to give knowledge an expanded meaning to include verbal information, numerical data, images, and imagery. Databases, computers, communications, and electronic devices will create a new generation of information. There is a *revolution* coming and nurse researchers must be a part of it! As stated previously, the new emphasis in health care is *accountability*. Data can help to improve quality of health care by identifying the most successful ways to treat conditions and identify areas that need improvement.

Thirty major managed-care health organizations (e.g., Kaiser Permanente, Blue Cross and Blue Shield, U.S. Health Care) have agreed to support the creation of a national data collection system that would produce a consumer "report card" on the quality of medical care in different hospital plans. The plans would be scored on their effectiveness in treating chronic illness, success rates for surgical operations, and patient satisfaction.

Developments in the 21st century include analysis of the human genome production of biological structure and function from genetic code, and rational drug design. These will require new and faster computers, advanced software, a National Research and Education Network, and expanded training of scientists in the use of computer-based tools. Health professionals need to have access to biomedical information made accessible through the higher performance computing technology and high-speed network resulting from High Performance Computing and Communications (HPCC) ("NLM Director," 1992).

High Performance Computing System (HPCS) is composed of four subcomponents: research for future generations of computing, system design tools, advanced prototype systems, and evaluation of early systems. HPCS will eventually be available in multiple architectures, many of which represent hybridizations of computational models used in earlier systems. New models of computation may yield higher performance for many classes of problems. A scaleable mass storage approach is now being used in most new high-performance computing systems. Operating system technology has been developed that is capable of supporting parallel and heterogeneous distributed applications of high-performance systems and workstations (Office of Science & Technology, 1992).

The use of interactive technology, expert systems, and electronic networking offers great potential for changes in health care delivery.

Databases, computers, communication and innovative electronic devices will create an entirely new *power* base of knowledge (information). The use of computerized data will help improve the quality of health care by identifying the most effective ways to treat patients' conditions. Nurse researchers must prepare for nursing research in the 21st century by developing and implementing a strategy that will make the best use of new technologies and methodologies.

Translating Science Into Public Health Policy

Science can help to identify health problems, suggest ways to control them, and help measure the results of decisions. As nursing research findings are translated into health policy, that which is scientific blends with that which is political. Public health policies emerge gradually and often in phases. Effective public health policy cannot be made without science, and health data and biomedical research are basic to science. Public health policy must be supported by a body of science so that *truth* can be convincingly determined (Taylor & Stith-Coleman, 1989).

References

Abdellah, F. G. (1957). Methods of identifying covert aspects of nursing problems. *Nursing Research, 6*, 4–23.

Abdellah, F. G. (1961). Criterion measures in nursing. *Nursing Research, 10*, 21–26.

Abdellah, F. G. (1970). *Overview of nursing research, 1955–1968*. Rockville, MD: National Center for Health Services Research and Development.

Abdellah, F. G. (1972). Evolution of nursing as a profession. *International Nursing Review, 19*, 219–235.

Abdellah, F. G. (1990). Research: Management of clinical trials. *Journal of Professional Nursing, 6*, 189.

Abdellah, F. G. (1991). *Nursing's role in the future: A case for health policy decision making*. Indianapolis, IN: Center Nursing Press of Sigma Theta Tau International.

Abdellah, F. G., Beland, I., Martin, A., & Matheney, R. (1960). *Patient centered approaches to nursing*. New York: Macmillan.

Abdellah, F. G., & Levine, E. (1954). *Appraising the clinical resources in small hospitals*. (USPHS No. 389.) Washington, DC: U. S. Government Printing Office.

Abdellah, F. G., & Levine, E. (1957a). Developing a measure of patient and personnel satisfaction with nursing care. *Nursing Research, 5*(3), 100–108.

Abdellah, F. G., & Levine, E. (1957b). *Patients and personnel speak: A method for studying patient care in hospitals* (Rev. 1964), (USPHS Pub. No. 527). Washington, DC: U. S. Government Printing Office.

Abdellah, F. G., & Levine, E. (1958). *Effect of nurse staffing on satisfaction with nursing care*. Chicago: American Hospital Association.

Abdellah, F. G., & Levine, E. (1986). *Better patient care through nursing research* (3rd ed.) New York: Macmillan.

Adams, M. E., McCall, N. T., Gray, D. T., Orza, M. J., & Chalmers, T. C. (1992). Economic analysis in randomized control trials. *Medical Care, 30*, 231–243.

Agency for Health Care Policy and Research. (1991). *Report to Congress: Progress of research on outcomes of health care services and procedures* (AHCPR Pub. No 91–0004). Rockville, MD: Author.

Agency for Health Care Policy and Research. (1992). *AHCPR-commissioned clinical practice guidelines*. Rockville, MD: Author.

Aiken, L. H. (Ed.) (1982). *Nursing in the 1980s: Crisis, opportunities, challenges*. Philadelphia: Lippincott.

Algase, D. L. (1992). Cognitive discriminants of wandering among nursing home residents. *Nursing Research, 41*, 78–81.

Amberson, J. B., Jr., McMahon, B. T., & Pinner, M. (1931). A clinical trial of sanocrysin in pulmonary tuberculosis. *American Review of Tuberculosis, 24*, 401–435.

American Nurses Association. (1980). *Nursing: a social policy statement* (Pub. No. NP-30). Kansas City, MO: Author.

American Nurses Association. (1989). Nursing's agenda calls for accessible care. *The American Nurse, 2*(1), 11.

American Nurses Association. (1991). *Standards of clinical nursing practice*. Kansas City, MO: Author.

American Nurses Association. (1992). *Nursing's agenda for health care reform*. Kansas City, MO: Author.

American Public Health Association. (1955, Nov. 16). News Release.

Anema, M., & Byrd, G. L. (1991). A systems model approach to increasing faculty productivity. *Journal of Nursing Education, 30*, 114–118.

Antman, E. M., Lau, J., Kupelnick, B., Mosteller, F., & Chalmers, T. C. (1992). A comparison of the results of meta-analyses of randomized control trials and recommendation of clinical experts. *Journal of the American Medical Association, 268*, 240–248.

Armitage, P. (1975). *Sequential medical trials* (2nd ed.). New York: John Wiley.

Arras, J. D. (1981). Health care vouchers and rhetoric of equity. *Hastings Center Report, 11*(4), 29–39.

Aspirin Myocardial Infarction Study Research Group. (1980). *Aspirin myocardial infarction study: Design, methods, and baseline results* (Pub. No. 80–2106). Washington, DC: U. S. Government Printing Office.

Atkinson, L. D., & Murray, M. E. (1983). *Understanding the nursing process* (2nd ed.) New York: Macmillan.

Aydelotte, M. K. (1962). The use of patient welfare as a criterion measure. *Nursing Research, 11,* 10–14.

Aydelotte, M. K. (1973). State of knowledge: nurse staffing methodology. In E. Levine (Ed.), *Report of the conference: Research on nurse staffing in hospitals 1972,* (pp. 7–13) (DHEW Pub, No. (NIH) 73–434.). Washington, DC: U. S. Government Printing Office

Aydelotte, M. K., & Tener, M. E. (1960). *An investigation of the relationship between nursing activity and patient welfare.* Washington, DC: U. S. Government Printing Office.

Bailar, J. C., Louis, T. A., Lavori, P. W., & Polanski, M. (1984). Studies without internal controls. *New England Journal of Medicine, 311,* 156–162.

Baker, B. (1993). Medical sleuths study older women—at last. *American Association for Retired People Bulletin, 34,* 4–5.

Baun, M. M. (1987). Doctoral preparation of qualified nurse researchers. *Research in Nursing and Health, 10* (3), iii–iv.

Benedict, R. (1934). *Patterns of culture.* New York: Penguin.

Benson, M. (1991, March 8). Health care: Overpriced, unjust—and unlikely to change. *St. Louis Post-Dispatch,* C1.

Bentley, J. (1992). Hospitals seek new ways to integrate health Care. *Hospitals, Journal of the American Hospital Association. 66,* 26–36.

Bernoulli, J. (1713). *Ars conjectandi (The art of conjecture).* Basle: University of Basle, Switzerland.

Block, D. (1990). Strategies for setting and implementing the national center for nursing research priorities. *Applied Nursing Research, 3,* 2–6.

Bloom, F. E., & Randolph, M. A. (Eds.) (1990). *Funding health sciences research: A strategy to restore balance.* Washington, DC: National Academy Press.

Bonuck, K. A. & Avno, P. S. (1993). What is access and what does it mean for nurses? In B. A. Kos-Munson (Ed.), *Who gets health care* (pp. 37–42). New York: Springer.

Brendenberg, V. C. (1951). *Nursing service research.* Philadelphia: Lippincott.

Brook, R. H., Davies-Avery, A., Greenfield, S., Harris, L. J., Lelah, T., Solomon, N. E., & Ware, J. E., Jr. (1977). Assessing the quality of medical care using outcome measures: An overview of the method. *Medical Care, 15* (Suppl. 9), 1–165.

Brooten, D. (1988). Effect of DRGs on research. In F. A. Shaeffer (Ed.) *Nursing Clinics of North America 23,* 587–596.

Brooten, D., Kumar, S., Brown, L. P., Butts, P., Finkler, A. A., Bakewell-Sachs, S., Gibbons, A., & Delivoria-Papadopoulos, M. (1986). A randomized clinical trial of early hospital discharge and home follow-up of very-low-birth-weight infants. *New England Journal of Medicine, 315,* 934–939.

Brown, A. A. (1991). Measurement of quality of primary studies for meta-analysis. *Nursing Research, 40,* 352–355.

Brown, A. A., & Grimes, D. E. (1993). Study shows nurse practitioner care may rival physician primary care. *American Nurse. 25*(2), 3.

Brown, D. (1992, August 10). Large, simple trials for big medical answers. *Washington Post,* p. A3.

Brown, E. L. (1948). *Nursing for the future.* New York: Russell.

Bryman, A. (1988). *Quantity and quality in social research.* London: Unwin.

Carey, R., & Posavec, E. (1978). Program evaluation of a physical medicine and rehabilitation unit: A new approach. *Archives of Physical Medicine and Rehabilitation, 59,* 330–337.

Cassidy, D. A., & Friesen, M. A. (1990). QA: Applying JCAHO's generic model. *Nursing Management, 21,* (6), 22–27.

Chiang, C. L. (1965). *An index of health: Mathematical models* (USPHS Pub. No. 1000). Washington, DC: U. S. Government Printing Office.

Clarke, L. (1992). Qualitative research: Meaning and language. *Journal of Advanced Nursing, 17,* 243–252.

Clinton, J. J., & Holohan, T. V. (1992). Technology assessment: Finding out what works. *Decisions in Imaging Economics, 5*(4), 12–16.

Cochran, W. G. (1937). Problems arising in the analysis of a series of similar experiments. *Journal of the Royal Statistical Society,*(Suppl 4), 102–118.

Cochran, W. G., & Cox, G. M. (1950). *Experimental designs.* New York: John Wiley.

Cohen, J. (1990). Things I have learned (so far). *American Psychologist, 45,* 1304–1312.

Cohen, M. R., & Nagel, E. (1934). *An introduction to logic and scientific method.* New York: Harcourt, Brace.

Cohn, V. (1992, September 15). Can managed care work? *The Washington Post.* pp. 10–11.

Cole, F. L., & Slocumb, E. M. (1990). Collaborative nursing research between novices: Productivity through partnership. *Nursing Forum, 25*(4), 13–18.

Committee for the Study of Nursing Education. (1923). *Nursing and nursing education in the United States.* New York: Macmillan.

Consensus Development Conference. (1985). Lowering blood cholesterol to prevent heart disease. *Journal of the American Medical Association, 253*, 2080–2086.

Cook, T. D., & Campbell, D. T. (1979). *Quasi-experimental designs for research in the field*. Chicago: Rand McNally.

Cooper, H., & Hedges, L. V. (Eds.). (1994). *The handbook of research synthesis*. New York:: Russel Sage Foundation.

Corman, L. C., & Davidson, R. A. (1992). Why clinical trials fail: The hidden assumptions of clinical trials. *Southern Medical Journal, 85*, 117–118.

Cordray, D. S. (1990). Strengthening causal interpretations of nonexperimental data: The role of meta-analysis. In L. Sechrest, E. Perrin, & J. Bunker (Eds.), *Research methodology: Strengthening causal interpretations of nonexperimental data* (pp. 151–172). (DHHS Publication No. (PHS) 90-3454). Rockville, MD: Agency for Health Care Policy and Research.

Crawford, E. D. (1992). Clinical trials: Conflicting opinions. *Journal of Urology, 148*, 387–388.

Crenshaw, A. B. (1991, February 24). Passing on retirement health costs. *Washington Post*, H1, H10.

Cronbach, L. J. (1970). *Essentials of psychological testing* (3rd ed.). New York: Harper & Row.

Curtin, L. (1986). Who says 'lean' must be 'mean'? *Nursing Management, 17*(1), 7–8.

David, J. A. (1982). Pressure sore treatment: A literature review. *International Journal of Nursing Studies, 19*, 183–191.

Davidhizar, R. E. (1988). Mentoring in doctoral education. *Journal of Advanced Nursing, 13*, 775–781.

Davis, A. R., Levine, E., & Sverha, S. (1986). *The national conference on nursing productivity: Report of the conference*. Washington, DC: Georgetown University.

Davis, C. K. (1993). Who will pay? the economic realities of health care reform. In B. A. Kos-Munson (Ed.), *Who gets health care* (pp. 43–45). New York: Springer.

Davis, G. C. (1988). Nursing values and health care policy. *Nursing Outlook, 36*, 289–292.

Deming, W. E. (1950). *Some theory of sampling*. New York: John Wiley.

Deming, W. E. (1975). On probability as a basis for action. *American Statistician, 29*, 146–152.

Dennis, K. E. (1991). Components of the doctoral curriculum that build success in the clinical nurse researcher role. *Journal of Professional Nursing, 7*, 160–175.

Denzin, N. K., & Lincoln, Y. S. (1994). *Handbook of qualitative research*. Thousand Oaks, CA: Sage.

Dickersin, K., Higgins, K., & Meinert, C. L. (1990). Identification of meta-analysis: The need for standard terminology. *Controlled Clinical Trials, 11*, 52–66.

Diers, D., & Burst, H. V. (1983). Effectiveness of policy related Research: Nurse-midwifery as case study. *Image, 15*, 68–74.

Dillon, W. R., & Goldstein, M. (1984). *Multivariate analysis: Methods and applications*. New York: John Wiley

Donabedian, A. (1966). Evaluating the quality of medical care. *Millbank Memorial Fund Quarterly, 44*, 166–206.

Donabedian, A. (1988). Quality and cost: Choices and responsibilities. *Inquiry, 25*, 90–99.

Donley, R. (1985). A social mandate for nursing: Prescription for the future. *Journal of Contemporary Health Law and Policy, 1*, 39–46.

Downs, F. S. (1978). Doctoral education in nursing: Future directions. *Nursing Outlook 26*, 56–61.

Downs, F. S. (1988). Doctoral education: Our claim to the future. *Nursing Outlook, 36*, 18–20.

Dracup, K. (1987). Critical care nursing. In J. J. Fitzpatrick & R. L. Taunton (Eds.), *Annual review of nursing research* Vol. 5, (pp. 107–133). New York: Springer Publishing Co.

Duke University Center for the Study of Aging (1978). *Multidimensional functional assessment: The OARS methodology* (2nd ed.). Durham, NC: Author.

Dunn, H. L. (1959). *The biological basis for high-level wellness*. Washington, DC: The Council for High Level Wellness.

Easterbrook, P. J. (1992). Directory of registries of clinical trials, *Statistics in Medicine, 11*, 345–359.

Edgeworth, F. Y. (1881). *Mathematical physics: An essay on the applications of mathematics to the moral sciences*. London: C. Kegan.

Edwards, J. N., Herman, J., Wallace, B. K., Pavy, M. D., & Harrison-Pavy, J. (1991). Comparison of patient-controlled and nurse-controlled anti-emetic therapy in patients receiving chemotherapy. *Research in Nursing and Health, 14*, 249–257.

Farren, E. A. (1991). Doctoral preparation and research productivity. *Nursing Outlook, 39*, 22–25.

Fechner, G. T. (1966). *Elements of psycho-physics*. (H. E. Adler, D. E. Hawes, & E. G. Boning, Trans.). New York: Holt, Rinehart and Winston, (Original work published 1860).

Fields, W. L. (1988). The PhD: The ultimate nursing doctorate. *Nursing Outlook, 36,* 188–189.

Fineberg, H. (1985). Future directions for research. *Medical Decision Making, 5*(1), 35.

Fisher, R. A. (1925). *Statistical methods for research workers.* Edinburgh: Oliver and Boyd.

Fisher, R. A. (1926). The arrangement of field experiments. *Journal of the Ministry of Agriculture of Great Britain, 33,* 503–513.

Fisher, R. A. (1935). *The design of experiments.* Edinburgh: Oliver and Boyd.

Fisher, R. A., (1947). *The design of experiments* (4th ed.). Edinburgh: Oliver and Boyd.

Fisher, R. A., & MacKenzie, W. A. (1923). Studies in crop variation. II: The manurial response of different potato varieties. *Journal of Agricultural Science, 13,* 311-320.

Fitzpatrick, J. J. (1987). The professional doctorate as an entry level into clinical practice. *NLN, 41*(2199), 53–56.

Fitzpatrick, J. J. (1992). Preface. In J. J. Fitzpatrick, R. L. Taunton, & A. K. Jacox (Eds.), *Annual Review of Nursing Research* (pp. vii–viii). *(10).* Springer Publishing Company.

Fitzpatrick, J. J., & Whall, A. L. (1983). *Conceptual models of nursing: Analysis and application.* Bowie, MD: Robert J. Brady.

Fitzpatrick, M. L. (1991). Doctoral preparation versus expectations. *Journal of Professional Nursing, 7,* 172–176.

Fleiss, J. L. (1986). *The design and analysis of clinical experiments.* New York: Wiley.

Flexner, A. (1925). *Medical education.* New York: Macmillan.

Friedman, L. M., Furberg, C. D., & DeMets, D. L. (1984). *Fundamentals of clinical trials.* Boston: John Wright.

Fry, V. S. (1953). The creative approach to nursing. *American Journal of Nursing, 53,* 301–302.

Fuller, E. O., Hasselmeyer, E. G., Hunter, J. C., Abdellah, F. G., & Hinshaw, A. S. (1991). Characteristics of the summary statements of the NIH nursing research applications. *Nursing Research, 40,* 346–351.

Gallant, B., & McLane, A. (1979). Outcome criteria: A process for validation at the unit level. *Journal of Nursing Administration, 9*,(1), 14–20.

Gehan, E. A., & Freireich, E. J. (1974). Non-randomized controls in cancer clinical trials. *New England Journal of Medicine, 290,* 198–203.

Geigle, R., & Jones, S. B. (1990). Outcomes measurement: A report from the front. *Inquiry, 17,* 7–13.

Ginsberg, G., Marks, I., & Waters, H. (1984). Cost-benefit analysis of a controlled trial of nurse therapy for neuroses in primary care. *Psychological Medicine, 14*, 683–690.

Giovannetti, P. (1978). *Patient classification systems in nursing: A description and analysis* (DHEW Pub. No. (HRA) 78–22). Springfield, VA: National Technical Information Service. (NTIS No. HRP–0500501)

Giovanetti, P., & Thiessen, M. (1983). *Patient classification for nurse staffing: Criteria for selection and implementation*. Edmonton, Alberta, Canada: Alberta Association of Registered Nurses.

Given, C. W., Given, B. A., & Coyle, B. W. (1985). Prediction of patient attrition from experimental behavioral interventions. *Nursing Research, 34*, 293–298.

Glaser, B. G., & Strauss, A. L. (1965). *Awareness of dying*. Chicago: Aldine.

Glaser, B. G., & Strauss, A. L. (1966). The purpose and credibility of qualitative research. *Nursing Research, 15*, 56–61.

Glaser, B. G., & Strauss, A. L. (1967). *Discovery of grounded theory: Strategies for qualitative research*. Chicago: Aldine.

Glass, G. V. (1976). Primary, secondary, and meta-analysis of research. *Educational Researcher, 5*, 3–18.

Glass, G. V., McGaw, B., & Smith, M. L. (1981). *Meta-analysis in social research*. Beverly Hills, CA: Sage.

Goldstein, J. (1992). Virginia Henderson Library leads nursing to new age. *Reflections, 18*, 9–11.

Goode, C. J., Titler, M., Rakel, B., Ones, D. S., Kleiber, C., Small, S., & Triolo, P. K. (1991). A meta-analysis of the effects of heparin flush and saline flush: Quality and cost implications. *Nursing Research, 40*, 324–330.

Goodwin, L. D., & Goodwin, W. L. (1984). Qualitative vs. quantitative research or qualitative and quantitative research? *Nursing Research, 33*, 378–380.

Grace, H. K. (1978). The development of doctoral education in nursing. *Journal of Nursing Education, 17*(4), 17–27.

Grace, H. K. (1989). Issues in doctoral education in nursing. *Journal of Professional Nursing, 5*, 266-270.

Grady, M. L. & Schwartz, H. A. (Eds.) (1993). *Automated data sources for ambulatory care effectiveness research*. Washington, DC: U. S. Government Printing Office.

Graunt, J. (1662). *Natural and political observations made upon the bills of mortality*. London: Roycroft.

Griffith, H. M. (1989). Historical perspectives and ANA policies. In ANA: *Classification system for describing nursing practice: Working papers* (pp. 4–5). Kansas City, MO: ANA

Griffith, H. M., Thomas, N., & Griffith, L. (1991). MDs bill for these routine nursing tasks. *American Journal of Nursing, 91,* (1), 22–26.

Grimes, D. A., & Schultz, K. F. (1992). Randomized controlled trials of home uterine activity monitoring: A review and critique. *Obstetrics and Gynecology, 79,* 137–142.

Guy, J. (1991). New challenges for nurses in clinical trials. *Seminars in Oncology Nursing, 7,* 297–302.

Guyatt, G., Sackett, D., Taylor, D. W., Chong, J., Roberts, R., & Pugsley, S. (1986). Determining optimal therapy-randomized trials in individual patients. *New England Journal of Medicine, 314,* 889–892.

Hahn, G. J., & Meeker, W. Q. (1993). Assumptions for statistical inference. *American Statistician, 47,* 1–11.

Hanchett, E. S. (1977). *The problem-oriented system: A literature review* (DHEW Pub. No. (HRA) 78–6). Springfield, VA: National Technical Information Service. (NTIS No. HRP–0500401)

Harmer, B., & Henderson, V. A. (1939). *Textbook of the principles and practices of nursing* (4th ed.). New York: Macmillan.

Hasselmeyer, E. G. (1961). *Behavior patterns of premature infants.* (US PHS Publication No. 840). Washington, DC: U. S. Government Printing Office.

Haussmann, R. K. D., & Hegyvary, S. T. (1977). *Monitoring quality of nursing care: Assessment and study of correlates* (DHEW Pub. No. (HRA) 77–70). Washington, DC: U. S. Government Printing Office.

Haygarth, J. (1800). *Of the imagination as a cause and as a cure of disorders of the body: Exemplified by fictitious tractors, and epidemical convulsions.* Bath, England: R. Cutwell.

Hedges, L. V., & Olkin, I. (1985). *Statistical methods for meta-analysis.* Orlando, FL: Academic Press.

Hendriksen, C., Lund, E., & Stromgard, E. (1984). Consequences of assessment and intervention among elderly people: A three year randomised controlled trial. *British Medical Journal, 289,* 1522–1524.

Hegyvary, S. T. (1986). Perspectives on nursing productivity: 1986. In A. R. Davis, E. Levine, & S. Sverha (Eds.), *The National Invitational Conference on Nursing Productivity.* Rockville, MD: National Center for Health Services Research (pp. 81–102).

Hegyvary, S. T., & Haussmann, R. D. (1976). Correlates of the quality of nursing care. *Journal of Nursing Administration, 6*(9), 22–27.

Hill, A. B. (1955). *Principles of medical statistics.* London: Lancet.

Hinshaw, A. S. (1988a). Research: Evolving clinical nursing research priorities: A national endeavor. *Journal of Professional Nursing, 4,* 398, 458–459.

Hinshaw, A. S. (1988b). Using research to shape health policy. *Nursing Outlook, 36*, 21–24.

Hinshaw, A. S., & Atwood, J. R. (1982). A patient satisfaction instrument: Precision by replication. *Nursing Research, 31*, 170–175.

Hoesing, H. & Kirk, R. (1990). Common sense quality management. *Journal of Nursing Administration, 20*(10), 10–15.

Holzemer, W. L., & Chambers, D. B. (1988). A contextual analysis of faculty productivity. *Journal of Nursing Education, 27*, 10–18.

Hover, J., & Zimmer, M. (1978). Nursing quality assurance: The Wisconsin system. *Nursing Outlook, 26*, 242–248.

Howland, D., & McDowell, W. E. (1964). The measurement of patient care: A conceptual framework. *Nursing Research, 13*, 4–7.

Hubbard, S. M. (1982). Cancer treatment research: The role of the nurse in clinical trials of cancer therapy. *Nursing Clinics of North America, 17*, 763–783.

Hudgings, C. (1990). *Library on line*. Indianapolis, IN: Sigma Theta Tau International.

Hughes, E. C., Hughes, H. M., & Deutscher, I. (1958). *Twenty thousand nurses tell their story*. Philadelphia: Lippincott.

Hunt, J. (1981). Indicators for nursing practice: The use of research findings. *Journal of Advanced Nursing, 6*, 189–194.

Hunter, J. E., & Schmidt, F. L. (1990). *Methods of meta-analysis*. Newbury Park, CA: Sage.

Institute of Medicine. (1988). *The future of public health*. Washington, DC: National Academy Press.

Institute of Medicine. (1990). *Summary. Forum on supporting biomedical research: Near-term problems and options for action*. Washington, DC: National Academy Press.

Jackson, G. B. (1978). *Methods for reviewing and integrating research in the social sciences: Final report to the National Science Foundation*. (Grant No. 76–20309) Washington, DC: Social Research Group, George Washington University.

Jelinek, R. C., & Dennis, L. C. (1976). *A review and evaluation of nursing productivity*. (DHEW, PHS. Pub. No. (HRA) 77–15.) Washington, DC: U. S. Government Printing Office.

Jelinek, R. C., Haussmann, R. K. D., Hegyvary, S. T., & Newman, J. F. Jr. (1974). *A methodology for monitoring quality of nursing care* (DHEW Pub. No. (HRA) 76–25). Washington, DC: U. S. Government Printing Office.

Jennings, B. M. (1991). Patient outcomes research: Seizing the opportunity. *Advanced Nursing Science, 14*, 59–72.

Jicks, T. D. (1979). Mixing qualitative and quantitative methods: Triangulation in action. *Administrative Science Quarterly, 24,* 602–611.

Johannessen, T., & Fosstvedt, D. (1991). Statistical power in single subject trials. *Family Practice, 8,* 384–387.

Johansen, M. A., Mayer, D. K., & Hoover, H. C. (1991). Obstacles to implementing cancer clinical trials. *Seminars in Oncology Nursing, 7,* 260–267.

Johns, E., & Pfefferkorn, B. (1934). *An activity analysis of nursing.* New York: Committee on the Grading of Schools of Nursing.

Johnson, J. E. (1993). Health care reform. *Nursing and Health Care, 14,* 59-60.

Joint Commission on the Accreditation of Healthcare Organizations (1988). *Guide to quality assurance.* Chicago: Author.

Joint Commission on the Accreditation of Healthcare Organizations (1990). *Accreditation manual for hospitals.* Chicago: Author.

Jones, E. W. (1974). *Patient classification for long-term care: User's manual* (DHEW Pub. No. HRA 75-3107). Washington, DC: U. S. Government Printing Office.

Kane, R. L., & Kane, R. A. (1981). *Assessing the elderly: A practical guide to management.* Lexington, MA: D. C. Heath.

Kannel, W. B., Neaton, J. D., Wentworth, D., Thomas, H. E., Stamler, J., Hulley, S. B., & Kjelsberg, M. O. (1986). Overall and CHD mortality rates in relation to major risk factors in 325,348 men screened for the MRFIT Multiple risk factor intervention trial. *American Heart Journal, 112,* 825–836.

Kaplan, A. (1964). *The conduct of inquiry.* New York: Chandler.

Katz, S., Ford, A. B., Moskowitz, R. W., Jackson, B. A., & Jaffee, M. W. (1963). Studies of illness in the aged: The index of ADL: A standardized measure of biological and psychosocial functioning. *Journal of the American Medical Association, 185,* 914–919.

Kazdin, A. E. (1992). *Methodological issues and strategies in clinical research.* Washington, DC: American Psychological Association.

Keohane, P. P., Jones, B. J. M., Attrill, H., Cribb, A., Northover, J., Frost, P., & Silk, D. B. A. (1983). Effect of catheter tunnelling and a nutrition nurse on catheter sepsis during parenteral nutrition. *Lancet, 2*(8364), 1388–1391.

Kessler, T. (1989). Research and policy formation: Is there a fit? *Journal of Professional Nursing, 5,* 246.

Ketefian, S. (1991). Doctoral preparation for faculty roles: Expectations and realities. *Journal of Professional Nursing, 7,* 105-11.

Kirpalani, H., Schmidt, B., McKibbon, K. A., Haynes, B., & Sinclair, J. C. (1989). Searching MEDLINE for randomized clinical trials involving care of the newborn. *Pediatrics, 83,* 543–546.

Knafl, K. A., & Breitmayer, B. J. (1991). Triangulation in qualitative research: Issues of conceptual clarity and purpose. In J. M. Morse (Ed.), *Qualitative nursing research: A contemporary dialogue* (pp. 226–239). Newbury Park, CA: Sage.

Kos-Munson, B. A. (Ed.). (1993). *Who gets health care?* New York: Springer Publishing Co.

Kraemer, H. C., & Thiemann, S. (1987). How many subjects? *Statistical power in research.* Newbury Park, CA: Sage.

Lachin, J. M. (1981). Introduction to sample size determination and power analysis for clinical trials. *Controlled Clinical Trials.* 2, 93–113.

Landsberger, H. A. (1958). *Hawthorne revisited.* Ithaca, NY: Cornell University.

Lang, N. M., & Dorman, K. (1990). The classification of patient outcomes. *Journal of Professional Nursing, 6,* 158–163.

Lawson, L.(1989). Developing investigators who will generate clinically relevant science. *Journal of Nursing Administration, 19*(1), 6–7.

Lawton, M. P. (1982). Competence, environmental pressure, and the adaptation of older people. In M. P. Lawton, P. G. Windley, & T. O. Byerts (Eds.), *Aging and the environment: Theoretical approaches* (pp. 33–59). New York: Springer.

Lawton, M. P. (1987). Behavioral and social components of functional capacity. In *Consensus development conference on geriatric assessment methods for clinical decisionmaking* (pp. 23–29). Bethesda, MD: National Institute on Aging.

Lawton, M. P., & Brody, E. M. (1969). Assessment of older people: Self-maintaining and instrumental activities of daily living. *Gerontologist, 9,* 179–186.

Lee, R. I., & Jones, B. (1933). *The fundamentals of good medical care.* Chicago: University of Chicago Press.

Le Fort, S. M. (1993). The statistical versus clinical significance debate. *Image, 25,* 57–62.

Leininger, M. M. (Ed.). (1985). *Qualitative research methods in nursing.* Orlando, FL: Grune.

Lembcke, P. A. (1956). Medical auditing by scientific methods. *Journal of the American Medical Association, 162,* 646–655.

Lenz, E. R. (1989). Doctoral faculty as a community of scholars: Positive environments for doctoral programs. *NLN, 15*(2238), 75–93.

Lenz, E. R., & Soeken, K. L. (1992). [Book Review of *Advanced nursing and health care research: Quantification approaches*]. *Nursing Science Quarterly, 5*, 94–95.

Levine, E. (1982). *The implications of the 1990 health objectives for the nation on health personnel supply and requirements: Final report to the Bureau of Health Professions.* Rockville, MD: Bureau of Health Professions.

Levine, E., & Abdellah, F. G. (1984). DRGs: A recent refinement to an old method. *Inquiry, 21*, 105–112.

Levine, E., Leatt, P., & Poulton, K. (1993). *Nursing practice in the UK and North America.* London: Chapman and Hall.

Lewis, F. M., Firsich, S. C., & Parsell, S. (1979). Clinical tool development for adult chemotherapy patients: Process and content. *Cancer Nursing, 2*, 99–108.

Liability—are you protected? (1991). *American Nurse, 23*(2), 33.

Lind, J. A. (1753). *A Treatise of the scurvy.* Edinburgh: Sands Murray and Cochran.

Light, R. J., & Pillemer, D. B. (1984). *Summing up: The science of reviewing research.* Cambridge, MA: Harvard University Press.

Lohr, K. N., (1989). Advances in health status assessment: Conference proceedings. *Medical Care, 27* (Suppl.), S1–S294.

Lohr, K. N., (1992). Advances in health status assessment: Fostering the application of health status measures in clinical settings. *Medical Care, 30* (Suppl.) MS1–MS294.

Louis, P. C. A. (1834). *Essay on clinical instruction.* London: S. Highley.

Louis, T. A., Lavori, P. W., Bailar, J. C., & Polansky, M. (1984). Crossover and self-controlled designs in clinical research. *The New England Journal of Medicine, 310*, 24–31.

Lynd, R. S. (1939). *Knowledge for what?* Princeton, NJ: Princeton University Press.

Lynd, R. S., & Lynd, H. M. (1929). *Middletown: A study in American culture.* New York: Harcourt Brace.

Macgregor, F. C. (1960). *Social science in nursing.* New York: Russell Sage Foundation.

MacIver, R. M. (1937). *Society: A textbook of sociology.* New York:Farrar and Rinehart.

Mallison, M. B. (1993). Nurses as house staff. *American Journal of Nursing. 93*(3), 7.

Mantel, N., & Haenszel, W. (1959). Statistical aspects of the analysis of data from retrospective studies of disease. *Journal of the National Cancer Institute, 22*, 719–748.

Maraldo, P. J. (1990). The nineties: A decade in search of meaning. *Nursing and Health Care, 11,* 11–14.

Marriner-Tomey, A. (1990) Historical development of doctoral programs from the Middle Ages to nursing education today. *Nursing & Health Care, 11,* 133–137.

Marshall, C., & Rossman, G. B. (1989). *Designing qualitative research.* Newbury Park, CA: Sage.

Martin, E. J., White, J. T., Hansen, M. (1989). Preparing students to shape health policy. *Nursing Outlook, 37,* 890–93.

Martin, M. J., Hulley, S. B., Browner, W. S., Kuller, L. H., & Wentworth, D. (1986). Serum cholesterol, blood pressure, and mortality: Implications from a cohort of 361,662 men. *Lancet, 2*(8513), 933-936.

Martinson, I. (1981). Nurse coordinated care of the child with advanced cancer. In L. Marino (Ed.), *Career Nursing* (pp. 431–440) St. Louis: Mosby.

Mason, R. L., Gunst, R. F., & Hess, J. L. (1989). *Statistical design and analysis of experiments.* New York: Wiley.

Matarazzo, J. D. & Abdellah, F. G. (1971). Doctoral education for nurses in the United States. *Nursing Research, 20,* 404–14.

Mayo, E. (1933). *The human problems of an individual civilization.* New York: Macmillan.

McCormick, K. A. (1988). Urinary incontinence in the elderly. *Nursing Clinics of North America, 23,* 135–137.

McCormick, K. A. (1992). Nursing effectiveness research using existing data bases. In National Center for Nursing Research, *Patient outcomes research: Examining the effectiveness of nursing practice.* Conference proceedings (pp. 203–209). (NIH Publication No. 93–3411) Bethesda, MD: National Institutes of Health

McGinnis, J. M., Richmond, J. B., Brandt, E. N., Windom, R. E., & Mason, J. O. (1992). Health progress in the United States: Results of the 1990 objectives for the nation. *Journal of the American Medical Association, 268,* 2545–2552.

Mead, M. (1939). *From the South Seas: Studies of adolescence and sex in primitive societies.* New York: William Morrow.

Megel, M. E., Langston, N. F. & Creswell, J. W. (1988). Scholarly productivity: A Survey of nursing faculty researchers. *Journal of Professional Nursing, 4,* 45–54.

Meinert, C. L., & Tonascia, S. (1986). *Clinical trials: Design, conduct, and analysis.* New York: Oxford University Press.

Meleis, A. I. (1988). Doctoral education in nursing. *Journal of Professional Nursing, 4,* 436–46.

Melink, T. J., & Whitacre, M. Y. (1991). Planning and implementing clinical trials. *Seminars in Oncology Nursing, 7*, 243–251.

Milio, N. (1984). Nursing research and the study of health policy. In H. H. Werley & J. J. Fitzpatrick (Eds.), *Annual Review of Nursing Research, 2*, (291–306). New York: Springer Publishing Co.

Miller, P., Wikoff, R., & Hiatt, A. (1992). Fishbein's model of reasoned action and compliance behavior of hypertensive patients. *Nursing Research, 41*, 104–109.

Mims, B. C. (1988). Development of clinical performance examination for critical care nurses. In O. L. Strickland & C. F. Waltz (Eds.), *Measurement of nursing outcomes: Measuring Nursing Performance Vol. 2* (pp. 96–108). New York: Springer Publishing Co.

Molde, S., & Diers, D. (1985). Nurse practitioner research: selected literature review and research agenda: *Nursing Research, 34*, 362–367.

Moore, D. S. (1985). *Statistics: Concepts and controversies* (2nd ed.). New York: W. H. Freeman.

Moritz, P. (1991). Innovative nursing practice models and patient outcomes. *Nursing Outlook, 39*, 111–114.

Morris, R. D., Audet, A., Angelillo, I. F., Chalmers, T. C., & Mosteller, F. (1992). Chlorination, chlorination by-products, and cancer: A meta-analysis. *American Journal of Public Health, 82*, 955–963.

Moses, E. (1990). *The registered nurse population: Findings from the national sample survey of registered nurses,* March 1988. Washington, DC U. S. Government Printing Office.

Moses, L. A. (1985). Statistical concepts fundamental to investigations. *New England Journal of Medicine, 312*, 890–897.

Mosteller, F. (1990). Improving research methodology: An overview. In L. Sechrest, E. Perrin, & J. Bunker (Eds.), *Research methodology: Strengthening causal interpretations of nonexperimental data* (DHHS Publication No. (PHS) 90-3454). Washington, DC: U. S. Government Printing Office.

Munhall, P., & Oiler, C. (1986). *Nursing research: A qualitative perspective.* Norwalk, CT: Appleton-Century Crofts.

Murdaugh, C. (1992). Quality of life, functional status, patient satisfaction. In, *Patient outcomes research: Examining the effectiveness of nursing practice.* (pp. 91–96). Washington, DC: U. S. Government Printing Office.

Murphy, J. F. (1985). Doctoral education of nurses: Historical development, programs, and graduates. In H. H. Werley & J. J. Fitzpatrick (Eds.), *Annual Review of Nursing Research 3*, (pp. 171–189). New York: Springer Publishing Co.

Murphy, N. J. (1992). Nursing leadership in health policy decision making. *Nursing Outlook, 40*, 158–161.

Murphy, S. A. (1989). Multiple triangulation applications in a program of nursing research. *Nursing Research, 38*, 294–298.

Naisbitt, J., & Aburdene, P. (1990). *Megatrends 2000. Ten new directions for the 1990s.* New York: William Morrow.

National Center for Nursing Research. (1989). *Facts about funding.* Bethesda, MD: Author.

National Center for Nursing Research. (1992a). *Facts about funding.* (NIH Publication No. 92–3112). Washington, DC: U. S. Government Office.

National Center for Nursing Research. (1992b). *Patient outcomes research: Examining the effectiveness of nursing practice.* (NIH Publication No. 93–3411.) Washington, DC: U. S. Government Printing Office.

National Center for Nursing Research. (1992c). *Research grants active in FY 1993.* Bethesda, MD: Author.

National Center for Nursing Research. (1992d). *Update: National Center for Nursing Research.* Bethesda, MD: Author.

National Institutes of Health. (1975). *NIH Inventory of clinical trials: Fiscal year 1975.* Bethesda, MD: NIH Division of Research Grants.

National Institutes of Health (1989). *Report of the 1989 NIH task force on nursing research.* (NIH Publication No. 89–487). Washington, DC: U. S. Government Printing Office.

National Institutes of Health (1992). *Framework for discussion of strategies for NIH.* Washington, DC: U. S. Government Printing Office.

National Institutes of Health. (1993). Preparing a research grant application to the *National Institute of Health.* Bethesda, MD: Author.

National League for Nursing Education (1937). *A study of nursing service in fifty selected hospitals.* New York: United Hospital Fund.

National League for Nursing Education. (1947). *A study of pediatric nursing.* New York: Author.

National League for Nursing Education. (1948). *A study of nursing service in one children's and twenty-one general hospitals.* New York: Author.

NLM director to head national office of high performance computing. (1992). *National Library of Medicine News, 47*(7–8), 11–12.

Nelson, N. M., Enkin, M. D., Saigal, S., Bennett, K. J., Milner, R., & Sackett, D. L. (1980). A randomized clinical trial of the Leboyer approach to childbirth. *New England Journal of Medicine, 302*, 655–660.

Newman, J. R. (1956). *The world of mathematics. Vol. 3*: New York: Simon and Schuster.

Newman, M. A. (1991). Health conceptualizations. In J. J. Fitzpatrick, R. L. Taunton, & A. K. Jacox (Eds.), *Annual Review of Nursing Research. (pp. 221–243)*. New York: Springer Publishing Co.

Nielsen, P. A. (1992). Quality of care: Discovering a modified practice theory. *Journal of Nursing Care Quality, 6*, 63–76.

Nightingale, F. (1858). *Notes on matters affecting the health efficiency, and hospital administration of the British army*. London: Harrison & Sons.

Nightingale, F. (1861). Hospital statistics and hospital plans. *Transactions of the National Association for the Promotion of Social Science, 4, 554–560*.

Norman, E., Gadaleta, D., & Griffin, C. C. (1991). An evaluation of three blood pressure methods in a stabilized acute trauma population. *Nursing Research, 40*, 86–89.

Nursing proposes health care reform. (1991). *American Nurse, 23*(2), 1.

Nutting, P. A. (1991). *A research agenda for primary care: Summary report of a conference*, Rockville, MD: Agency for Health Care Policy and Research.

Nyamanthi, A. M., Leake, B., Flaskerud, J., Lewis, C., & Bennett, C. (1993). Outcomes of AIDs counseling programs for impoverished women of color. *Research in Nursing and Health, 16*, 11–20.

O'Brien-Pallas, L., Cockerill, R., & Leatt, P. (1992). Different systems, different costs? An examination of the comparability of workload measurement systems. *Journal of Nursing Administration, 22*(12), 17–22.

Office of Science and Technology Policy. (1992). *Grand challenges 1993: High performance computing and communications: The FY 1993 U. S. research and development program*. Washington, DC: U. S. Government Printing Office.

O'Hare, P. (1992). Comparing two models of discharge planning rounds. *Applied Nursing Research, 5*, 66–73.

Olds, D. L., Henderson, C. R. Jr., Tatelbaum, R., & Chamberlin, R. (1986). Improving the delivery of prenatal care and outcomes of pregnancy: A randomized trial of nurse home visitation. *Pediatrics, 77*, 16–28.

O'Malley, M. N., & Kossack, C. F. (1950). A statistical study of factors influencing the quality of patient care in hospitals. *American Journal of Public Health, 40*, 1428–1432.

O'Neil, E. H. (1993). *Health professions education for the future*. In *Service to the nation* (pp. 83–90). San Francisco, CA: PEW Health Profession Commission.

Palmer, R., H. Donabedian, A., & Povar, G. J. (1991). *Striving for quality in health care: An inquiry into policy and practice*. Ann Arbor, MI. Health Administration Press.

Parse, R., Coyne, A. B., & Smith, M. J. (1985). *Nursing research: Qualitative methods.* Bowie, MD: Brady Communications.

Patton, M. Q. (1990). *Qualitative evaluation and research methods.* Newbury Park, CA: Sage.

Pearson, K. (1896). Regression, heredity, and panmixia. *Philosophical Transactions of the Royal Society, 187A,* 253–258.

Pearson, K. (1904). Report on certain enteric fever inoculation statistics. *British Medical Journal, 2,* 1243–1246.

Pender, N. J. (1992a). Reforming health care: Future Directions. *Nursing Outlook, 40,* 8–9.

Pender, N. J. (1992b). The NIH strategic plan: How will it affect the future of nursing science and practice. *Nursing Outlook, 41,* 55–56.

Pepper Commission (1990). *A call for action. The Pepper Commission on comprehensive health care.* Executive Summary. Washington, DC, U. S. Government Printing Office.

Perlow, M. (1988). The Perlow self-esteem scale. In O. L. Strickland & CF. Waltz (Eds.), *Measurement of nursing outcomes* (pp. 135–143). New York: Springer.

Pfefferkorn, B. (1932). Measuring nursing, quantitatively and qualitatively. *American Journal of Nursing, 32,* 80–85.

Pfefferkorn, B., & Rovetta, C. A. (1940). *Administrative cost analysis for nursing service and nursing education.* New York: National League for Nursing Education.

Phaneuf, M. (1976). *The nursing audit* (2nd ed.). New York: Appleton-Century-Crofts.

Plan calls for health care reform. (1991b). *American Nurse, 23,* 1, 8, 17.

Popovsky, M. D., & Ilstrup, D. M. (1986). Randomized clinical trial of transparent polyurethane IV. dressings. *NITA, 9,* 107–110.

Pranulis, M. F. (1985). Researchmanship: Characteristics of productive research environments in nursing. *Western Journal of Nursing Research, 7,* 127–31.

Rabenek, L., Viscoli, C. M., & Horwitz, R. I. (1992). Problems in the conduct and analysis of randomized clinical trials. *Archives of Internal Medicine, 152,* 507–512.

Raymond, C. A. (1986). Can fewer patients, studied more intensively, solve historic problems of MS clinical trials? *Journal of the American Medical Association, 256,* 691–692.

Reiter, F., & Kokosh, M. E. (1963). *Quality of nursing care: Report of a field study to establish criteria, 1950–1954.* New York: Columbia University, Institute of Research and Studies in Nursing Education.

Reynolds, N. R., Timmerman, G., Anderson, J., & Stevenson, J. S. (1992). Meta-analysis for descriptive research. *Research in Nursing and Health, 15*, 467–475.

Rice, F. A. (1987). The role of the nurse in health care management at policy-making level. *World of Irish Nursing, 16*(1), 5–7.

Rich, S. (1991, March 14). 35 million Americans seen limited by disabilities. *The Washington Post*, A10.

Ripsin, C. M., Keenan, J. M., Jacobs, D. R., Elmer, P. J., Welcher, R. R., Van Horn, L., Lui, K., Turnbull, W. H., Thye, F. W., Kestin, M., Hegsted, M., Davidson, D. M., Davidson, M. H., Dugan, L. D., Demark-Wahnefried, W., & Beling, S. (1992). Oat products and lipid lowering. *Journal of the American Medical Association, 267*, 3317–3325.

Roethlisberger, F. J., & Dickson, W. J. (1939). *Management and the worker*. Cambridge, MA: Harvard University.

Rogers, M. E. (1970). *An introduction to the theoretical basis of nursing*. Philadelphia: Davis.

Rooks, J. P. (1990). Let's admit we ration health care—then set priorities. *American Journal of Nursing, 90*(6), 39–43.

Sampselle, C. M., & DeLancey, J. O. L. (1992). The urine stream interruption test and pelvic muscle function. *Nursing Research, 41*, 72–76.

Schwartz, D., Henley, B., & Zeitz, L. (1964). *The elderly ambulatory patient: Nursing and psycho-social needs*. New York: Macmillan.

Sechrest, L., & Hannah, M. (1990). The critical importance of nonexperimental data. In L. Sechrest, E. Perrin, & J. Bunker (Eds.), *Research methodology: Strengthening causal interpretations of nonexperimental data*. (pp. 1–7). (DHHS Pub. No. (PHS) 90–3454). Rockville, MD: Agency for Health Care Policy and Research. (NTIS No. PB90–101387).

Selltiz, C., Wrightsman, L. S., & Cook, S. W. (1976). *Research methods in social relations* (3rd ed.). New York: Holt, Rinehart and Winston.

Sheps, M. C. (1955). Approaches to quality of hospital care. *Public Health Reports, 70*, 877–886.

Sherwen, L. N., Bevil, C. A., Adler, D., & Watson, P. G. (1993). Educating for the future: A national survey of nursing deans about need and demand for nurse researchers. *Journal of Professional Nursing, 9*, 195–203.

Shewhart, W. A. (1931). *Economic control of quality of manufactured product*. New York: Van Nostrand.

Shumaker, S. A., Schron, E. B., & Ockene, J. K. (Eds.). (1990). *The handbook of health behavior change*. New York: Springer Publishing Co.

Sigma Theta Tau International, (1986). Ten-year plan for knowledge. Indianapolis, IN: Author.

Sigma Theta Tau International. (1992). *Virginia Henderson International Nursing Library: The electronic library*. Indianapolis, IN: Author.

Simmons, L. W., & Henderson, V. (1964). *Nursing research: A survey and assessment*. New York: Appleton-Century-Crofts.

Simmons, L. W., & Wolff, G. (1954). *Social Science in Medicine*. New York: Russell Sage.

Simon, J. R. (1961). Nurses' ratings of patient welfare as criterion measures in the health sciences. *Occupational Psychology, 35*, 10–22.

Siu, A. L., Manning, W. G., & Benjamin, B. (1990). Patient, provider, and hospital characteristics associated with inappropriate hospitalization. *American Journal of Public Health, 80, 1253–1256*.

Smith, G. (1988). Speaker urges nurses to move health agenda. *American Nurse, 20*(10), 25.

Smith, M. C. (1988). *Meta-analysis of nursing research*. Birmingham, AL: Author.

Social Security Amendments of 1972, P. L. 92–603.

Spilker, B. (1986). *Guide to clinical interpretation of data*. New York: Raven Press.

Starr, P. (1992). *The logic of health—care reform*. Knoxville, TN: The Grand Rounds Press.

Stevens, P. E. (1993). Who gets care? Access to health care as an arena for nursing action. In B. A., Kos-Munson. (Ed.), *Who gets health care*. (p. 11). New York: Springer.

Stevenson, J. S. (1992). Review of the first decade of the annual review of nursing research. In J. J. Fitzpatrick, R. L. Taunton, & A. K. Jacox (Eds.), *Annual Review of Nursing Research*, (Vol. 10, pp. 1–22). New York: Springer Publishing Co.

Stewart, A. L., Ware, J. E. Jr., & Brook, R. H. (1982). *Construction and scoring of aggregate functional status measures*. (Report No. R–2551–1–HHS). Santa Monica, CA: Rand Corporation.

Stewart, B. J., & Archbold, P. G. (1992). Focus on psychometrics: Nursing intervention studies require outcome measures that are sensitive to change: Part I. *Research in Nursing and Health, 15*, 477–481.

Stewart, B. J., & Archbold, P. G. (1993). Focus on psychometrics: Nursing intervention studies require outcome measures that are sensitive to change: Part II. *Research in Nursing and Health, 16*, 77–81.

Stichele, R. V. (1991). Measurement of patient compliance and the interpretation of randomized clinical trials. *European Journal of Clinical Pharmacology, 41*, 27–35.

Stouffer, F. A., Suchman, E. A., DeVinney, L. C., Star, S. A., & Williams, R. M. (1949–1950). *Studies in social psychology in World War II*. Vols 1–4. Princeton, NJ: Princeton University Press.

Strauss, A. (1963). *Hospital personnel, nursing care and dying patients*. San Francisco, CA: University of California.

Strauss, A. (1987). *Qualitative analysis for social scientists*. New York: Cambridge University Press.

Strauss, A., & Corbin, J. (1990). *Basics of qualitative research: Grounded theory procedures and techniques*. London: Sage.

Strauss, S. S. (1988). Information preference and information seeking in hospitalized surgery patients In C. F. Waltz & O. L. Strickland (Eds.), *Measurement of nursing outcomes: Vol. 1*: Measuring client outcomes (pp. 61–79). New York: Springer Publishing Co.

Strickland, O. L., & Waltz, C. F. (Eds.). (1988). *Measurement of nursing outcomes: Vol 2: Measuring nursing performance: Practice, education, and research;* New York: Springer Publishing Co.

Strickland, O. L., & Waltz, C. F. (Eds.). (1990), *Measurement of nursing outcomes: Vol 4: Measuring client self-care and coping skills;* New York: Springer Publishing Co.

Stuart, A., & Ord, J. K. (1991). *Kendall's advanced theory of statistics: Vol. 2:* Classical inference and relationships (5th ed.). New York: Oxford University Press.

Sullivan, D. F. (1966). *Conceptual problems in developing an index of health*. (DHEW Pub. No. (HRA) 74–1017). Washington, DC: U. S. Government Printing Office.

Tannock, I. F. (1992). Some problems related to the design and analysis of clinical trials. *International Journal of Radiation Oncology, Biology, & Physics, 22*, 881–885.

Taylor, S. E. & Stith-Coleman, I. (1989). Translating Science into Public Health Promotion. In *CRS Review: Public Health Policy and the Congress*. Washington, DC: Congressional Research Service.

Thompson, S. G., & Pocock, S. J. (1991). Can meta-analysis be trusted? *Lancet, 338*, 1127–1130.

Thornquist, M. D., Patrick, D. L., & Omenn, G. S. (1991). Participation and adherence among older men and women recruited to the beta-carotene and retinol efficacy trial (CARET). *Gerontologist, 31*, 593–597.

Tilden, V. P., Nelson, C. A., & May, B. A. (1990). Use of qualitative methods to enhance content validity. *Nursing Research, 39*, 172–175.

Tippett, L. H. C. (1931). *The method of statistics*. London: Williams and Norgate.

U. S. Department of Health, Education and Welfare. (1971). *Extending the scope of nursing practice*. Washington, DC: U. S. Government Printing Office.

U. S. Department of Health and Human Services. (1986). *Surgeon general's workshop on violence and public health report*. (DHHS Publication No. HRS–D–MC 86–1). Washington, DC: U. S. Government Printing Office.

U. S. Department of Health and Human Services. (1990). *Promoting health, preventing disease: Year 2000 objectives for the nation*. Washington, DC: U. S. Government Printing Office.

U. S. Department of Health and Human Services. (1991). *Healthy people 2000: National health promotion goals and disease prevention objectives* (USDHHS Pub. No. (PHS) 91–50212). Washington, DC: U. S. Government Printing Office.

U. S. Department of Health and Human Services, National Center for Health Statistics. (1992). *Health United States 1991 and prevention profile* (DHHS Pub. No. (PHS) 92–1232). Washington, DC: U. S. Government Printing Office.

U. S. Department of Health, Education, and Welfare, Division of Nursing Resources. (1954). *How to study nursing activities in a patient unit*. (US PHS Pub. No. 370). Washington, DC: U. S. Government Printing Office.

U. S. Department of Health, Education, and Welfare, Public Health Service (1979). *Healthy people: The surgeon general's report on health promotion and disease prevention*. DHEW (PHS) Pub. No. 79–55071. Washington, DC: U. S. Government Printing Office.

U. S. General Accounting Office. (1992). *Cross design synthesis: A new strategy for medical effectiveness research* (GAO/PEMD–92–18). Washington, DC: Author.

Urinary Incontinence Guideline Panel. (1992). *Urinary incontinence in adults*. (AHCPR Pub. No. 92–0038). Rockville, MD: Agency for Health Care Policy and Research.

Valinsky, D. (1975). Simulation. In L. J. Shuman, R. D. Speas, Jr., & J. P. Young (Eds.), *Operations research in health care* (pp. 144–176). Baltimore: Johns Hopkins University Press.

Van Amringe, M., & Shannon, T. F. (1992). Awareness, assimilation, and adoption: The challenge of effective dissemination. *Quality Review Bulletin, 18*, 397–404.

Vehvilainer-Julikunen, K. (1992). Client-public health nurse relationships in child health care: A grounded-theory study. *Journal of Advanced Nursing, 17*, 896–904.

Volicer, B. J. (1984). *Multivariate statistics for nursing research*. Orlando, FL: Grune and Stratton.

Wade, D. T., Langton-Hewer, R., Skilbeck, C. E., Bainton, D., & Burns-Cox, C. (1985). Controlled trial of a home-care service for acute stroke patients. *Lancet, 1*(8424), 323–327.

Wahrendorf, J., & Blettner, M. (1985). An investigation of the adequacy of randomization. *Controlled Clinical trials, 6,* 249–258.

Walker, E. (1992). *Annotated bibliography: Quality-of-care research.* (AHCPR Pub. No. 92–0029). Washington, DC: U. S. Government Printing Office.

Wallis, W. A., & Roberts, H. V. (1965). *The nature of statistics.* New York: The Free Press.

Waltz, C. F., & Strickland, O. L. (Eds.) (1988). *Measurement of nursing outcomes: Vol 1: Measuring client outcomes:* New York: Springer Publishing Co.

Waltz, C. F., & Strickland, O. L. (Eds.). (1990). *Measurement of nursing outcomes: Vol 3: Measuring clinical skills and professional development in education and practice:* New York: Springer Publishing Co.

Wandelt, M. A., & Aga, J. W. (1974). *Quality patient can scale.* New York: Appleton-Century-Crofts.

Wandelt, M. A., & Stewart, D. S. (1975). *Slater nursing competencing rating scale.* New York: Appleton-Century-Crofts.

Ward, M. J., & Lindeman, C. A. (1978). *Instruments for measuring nursing practice and other health variables* (DHEW Pub. No. HRA 78–53). Washington, DC: U. S. Government Printing Office.

Ware, J. E. (1976). Scales for measuring general health perceptions. *Health Services Research, 2,* 396–415.

Weed, L. L. (1964). Medical records, patient care, and medical education, *Irish Journal of Medical Science, 6,* 271–282.

Wenger, N. K., Mattson, M. E, Furberg, C. D., & Elinson, J. (Eds.), (1984). *Assessment of quality of life in clinical trials of cardiovascular therapies.* New York: LeJacq.

Werley, H. H., & Lang, N. M. (1988). *Identification of the nursing minimum data set.* New York: Springer Publishing Co.

White, K. L. (1974). Health information and the nation's health. In V. Saba & E. Levine (Eds.), *Management information systems for public health/community health agencies: Report of the conference* (pp. 17–28). New York: National League for Nursing.

White, R. M. (1991). The ending frontier: Too many researchers, too few dollars. *Issues in Science and Technology, 7*(3), 35–37.

Willems, Y. (1990). Cancer research and the research nurse. *Nursing Standard, 5*(6), 30–32.

Williams, B. S. (1986). Career development of the nurse-scientist: the new doctorate faces a postdoctoral. *Journal of Professional Nursing, 4*, 73.

Williams, B. S. (1988). The challenge to black nurses. *Journal of National Black Nurses Association, (2)*, 11–15.

Williams, C. A. (1989). Doctoral programs in nursing and the development of research centers. *Journal of Professional Nursing, 5*, 117,168.

Williams, R. & Blackburn, R. T. (1988). Mentoring and junior faculty productivity. *Journal of Nursing Education, 27*, 204–209.

Wilson, H. S. (1991). Identifying problems for clinical research to create a nursing tapestry. *Nursing Outlook, 39*, 280–282.

Wondoloski, C. (1991). The lived experience of health in the oldest old: A phenomenological study. *Nursing Science Quarterly, 4*, 113–118.

World Health Organization. (1978). *Primary health care: Report of the international conference on primary health care, Alma Ata, USSR.* Geneva: Author.

World Health Organization. (1984). *List of proposed indicators for monitoring progress towards health for all in the European region* (Report No. EUR/RC34/13 4762D/265OD). Copenhagen: Author.

Wyszewianski, L. (1988). Quality of care: Past achievements and future challenges. *Inquiry, 25*, 13–22.

Yura, H., & Walsh, M. (1978). *The nursing process: Assessing, planning, implementing, evaluating* (3rd ed.). New York: Appleton-Century Crofts.

Zelen, M. (1969). Play the winner rule and the controlled clinical trial. *Journal of the American Statistical Association, 64*, 131–146.

Index

SP *Springer Publishing Company*

JOURNAL OF NURSING MEASUREMENT

JOURNAL

Editors: **Ada Sue Hinshaw,** PhD, RN, FAAN, and **Ora L. Strickland,** PhD, RN, FAAN

The *Journal of Nursing Measurement,* is the only journal that specifically addresses instrumentation in nursing. It serves as a forum for disseminating information on instruments, tools, approaches, and procedures developed or utilized for measuring variables in nursing. The editorial team unites two of the leading nurses in the field: Ora Strickland, who coedits the landmark volumes *Measurement of Nursing Outcomes,* and Ada Sue Hinshaw, one of the nation's leading nurse researchers.

The *Journal of Nursing Measurement* is a refereed publication. Articles are reviewed by members of the editorial board, comprised of measurement experts with backgrounds in a variety of clinical and functional areas. Each manuscript is reviewed by at least two authorities on the topic, ensuring reliable material in each and every issue.

Sample Contents:

"Measurement of Mealtime Interactions Among Persons with Dementing Disorders," by Linda R. Phillips, Ph.D., R.N., F.A.A.N. and Suzanne Van Ort, Ph.D., R.N., F.A.A.N.

"Development of the Stimulus Intensity Modulation Scale," by Janet L. Blenner, Ph.D., R.N.

"A Quantitative Survey to Measure Energy Expenditure in Mid-life Women," by JoEllen Wilbur, Ph.D., R.N.,C; Karyn Holm, Ph.D., R.N., F.A.A.N. and Alice Dan, Ph.D.

"Measurement of Functional Ability in Patients with Coronary Artery Disease," by Patricia Keresztes, MS., R-N, C.C.F.N., Karyn Holm, Ph.D., R.N., F.A.A.N., Sue Penckofer, M.S., R.N., and Sharon Merritt, E.D., R.N.

(2 issues annually) • *ISSN 1061-3749*

536 Broadway, New York, NY 10012-3955 • (212) 431-4370 • Fax (212) 941-7842

⑤ *Springer Publishing Company*

ESSENTIALS OF NURSING RESEARCH, *5th Edition*

Lucille E. Notter, RN, EdD, FAAN, and
Jacqueline R. Hott, RN, CS, PhD, FAAN

Praise for earlier edition:

"The impressive credentials and rich clinical experience of the authors, combined with their flair for simplifying complex material, enables practice-based scientific inquiry to virtually come alive in these pages ... A winsome 'how-to' manual that will spark the intellectual curiosity and spirit of inquiry in nursing's bright young professionals."

—Nursing Research

Contents:

I. Introduction to Research. Evolution of the Research Movement in Nursing • The Meaning and Purpose of Research

II. The Research Process. Selecting a Problem • The Literature Search • The Hypothesis • The Research Method • Data Collection • Analysis of the Data • Findings, Conclusions, and Recommendations • The Research Report: Communicating the Findings

III. Evaluation of Research. The Evaluation Process

1994   224pp   0-8261-1598-5   softcover

536 Broadway, New York, NY 10012-3955 • (212) 431-4370 • Fax (212) 941-7842